ALOE
Myth
Magic
Medicine

ALOE
Myth
Magic
Medicine

Library of Congress Catalog Card
No. 89-050558

ISBN 1-878491-00-8

First edition, first printing, June, 1989

First edition, second printing, February, 1990

DEDICATION

This book is dedicated to my patient and understanding wife, Jessica Lockerd Hennessee, and to my daughters, Lauren and Mikel, who spent many evenings alone because of my work. It is also lovingly dedicated to the determined and untiring efforts of my mother Edna Miller Hennessee, and to the memory of Dewayne Kann and George Shoff. I express my appreciation to those who have freely shared their experience, knowledge, and valuable time...you know who you are.

ACKNOWLEDGMENTS

The final preparation of any book is always a formidable undertaking which involves many people. First, I must thank Bill R. Cook and Marilyn S. Krebs for their insight, which helped formulate my thought into a workable manuscript. Many thanks are due to Slada Lewis for assistance in confirming the chemistry of the Aloe vera plant, and to Glenn Freeman, Pat Terry and Arneta Lockerd for proofing the final work as well as Brad Buttry and Norman Tippeconnie for the typesetting and final preparation of the maps, pictures and graphic design of the texts.

CONTENTS

The Overselling of Aloe Vera
Standards -N.A.S.C.

FORWARD

During the course of writing this book, I have shared my thoughts with many people whom I respect. Many friends have encouraged me to fill the book with amazing testimonials, believing that such a book would be more appealing to the consumer. Some of my friends in the medical world have encouraged me to produce a work which is strictly medical in nature, believing that such a book would open the minds of medicine to the benefits of Aloe. Some think I should say nothing here that might offend either group. Finally, one or two individuals have discouraged me from making any reference to my personal, religious beliefs.

Although I am, of course, willing to listen to advice, I have, ultimately, pursued the course I originally set for myself and this book--to honestly review the historical and scientific evidence concerning Aloe vera and to pass along my experience concerning the economic realities of growing and producing Aloe products for the consumer. I have steadfastly refused to relate the healing effects of Aloe vera unless I have personally witnessed them. My religious beliefs are part of my personal philoshophy for which I make no apologies. Without my faith in Jesus Christ, this book would not exist, for without the strength given me by that faith, I would have quit this battle long ago.

Odus M. Hennessee

INTRODUCTION

Our present emerging state of holistic health consciousness is due in part to people like Odus Hennessee, who are
willing to look beyond traditional thinking in health care.

An open mind among health professionals is only one
stage in the wholistic health movement. The education of the
patient is also paramount in the new health consciousness.
This is the day of individuals being responsible for themselves and their health expression.

Information is the key to knowledge. In Myth, Magic,
Medicine, Odus Hennessee communicates his vast
knowledge along with the most current Aloe vera research,
making this book the definitive text about the Aloe vera plant
and its properties--mythical, magical, or medicinal.

Bill Wolfe, D.D.S., P.A.

PART I

MYTH

CHAPTER ONE

SEARCH FOR TRUTH

Spencer, the English poet wrote:

"There is a principle which is a bar against all information, which is proof against all argument and cannot help but keep man in everlasting ignorance, which is condemnation without investigation."

To paraphrase Spencer:

"There is a principle which has been applied to Aloe vera --Elaboration without investigation reaches its own level of condemnation."

This book represents an on-going investigation exploring the mysteries of Aloe vera and the often misunderstood world of plants. This exploration will continue for years to come as the contents of the book are read around the world by medical professionals and laypersons alike, all possessing one trait in common -- the search for truth.

Although God's truth be absolute...man's understanding of it is not. This understanding, as with all things in nature, is by degrees...shades of grey...tell me what is black and what is white...what is right and what is wrong...what is legal and what is illegal...and by whose definition, God's or man's? Is truth a matter of geography; is it okay to perform an act or service; on this side of the river or county line but not okay on the other side; is it legal on this side of the road but illegal across the road, just because it crosses a state line?

Is truth a matter of time, according to a man-made test? Does mere time contain within itself, the ability to change right to wrong or wrong to right, according to changing times? We think not. However, we know "truth" changes according to man's interpretation and level of knowledge, and, as such, is never constant. Perhaps change is the only absolute.

Does the adage, "Nothing is either good nor bad, but believing makes it so," hold true--as Shakespeare wrote, attempting to make sense out of chaos? We think not. What degree of truth can be comprehended, can be found within the human mind. It is all a state of mind...it is hidden within each individual's attitude, his attitude toward self...toward others...toward nature....and toward God. Each of us carries within us fragments of truth which, when combined, forms our whole (or total or absolute) truth. So, it profits us to strive to learn for ourselves that we may move toward God's perfection. No man is perfect except Jesus, but each of us has within us a seed of God which must be nurtured.

Our search for truth within the world of the Aloe vera has taken us down many roads. A price has been paid and will continue to be paid for experience. On occasion, we have encountered unmarked dead end streets and cul-de-sacs, and on occasion, we have collided with on-coming theories or hypotheses which have shattered ideas which we held to be true, simply because the idea came from an authority, expert, or source from which we acquired our first information. To separate the Myth, Magic, and Medicine of Aloe vera is almost as difficult as attempting to separate the gel, sap, and rind of the actual plant.

Scientific studies have proven that the most effective use of Aloe vera comes with a balanced blend of all three...the gel, the sap, and the rind. The gel plays its role when mixed properly with the sap but has little medical value alone. The sap contains most of the medical agents and is much more than just a purgative or treatment for minor skin injuries. The outer rind has appeared virtually worthless to some, but it, also, contains medical agents and many of the same nutrients found in the sap and the gel. Furthermore, chemical studies show that the rind is neither harmful nor dangerous as some have stated. Evidence suggests that the most effective use of the plant is to use the whole leaf.

Myths about the Aloe vera have been grafted onto ancient knowledge about the plant. Over the centuries, Aloe has been dressed in a veil of fiction which has contaminated the plant as a field of scientific study. The Aloe vera plant does some amazing things; this is a fact. However, over the years, opportunistic individuals have replaced facts with a jumble of half-truths and distortions which have tainted the truth about this wonderful plant with the unwelcome status of sheer magic. Some promoters of Aloe vera have used distorted historical references, individual testimonials, and fragments of medical reports to promote the gel alone as a healing agent and cure-all.

Much information is available about Aloe vera, but information alone is not sufficient to mirror truth. Truth comes only when information is transformed into knowledge and when this knowledge is blended with one's own personal experience and the results tested in the laboratory of the mind. Thus, we produce a distillation called wisdom, and, only then, can we hope to approach the throne of God's truth.

In this book we have attempted to separate Myth, Magic and Medicine just as laboratories have separated the component parts of the Aloe vera leaf in an attempt to understand its properties.

CHAPTER TWO

MIRACLE PLANT?

All over the world today, Aloe vera is a common household plant. It is, without doubt, one of the most talked about, yet most misunderstood, medical plants in history.

Most botanists agree, and historical evidence indicates that the plant originated in the warm, dry climates of Africa. But today the plant is found world-wide. Transplanted by man, it has adapted itself so successfully that it is found growing wild in many warm lands.

Although Aloe vera is a tropical plant, the root will survive freezing air temperatures as long as the ground does not freeze. When this happens, the leaves will be destroyed, but small plants (pups or suckers) will re-grow from the root. This occurred in the winter of 1983-84, one of the coldest in United States history, when at least ninety-six per cent of the Aloe vera growing in the Rio Grande Valley of Texas was destroyed. Some four to five thousand acres were devastated. Today, less than one thousand acres have been re-planted. However the plant does not have to freeze for the leaves to be damaged. Some loss of nutrients occurs below forty (40) degrees Fahrenheit and severe nutrient loss occurs at temperatures below thirty-five (35) degrees.

Conversely, Aloe vera will grow at 120 degrees Fahrenheit and can survive at much higher temperatures. It can survive extended droughts, going many months without water, yet it will thrive in the jungle as long as the root does not stand in water which drowns the plant.

The virtues of Aloe vera have been recorded by many ancient civilizations, including those of Persia, Egypt, Greece, Italy, India, and Africa. In modern times the plant is mentioned in the folklore of the Philippines and the islands of Southeast Asia including Malaysia. It is known in Tahiti, Japan, and Hawaii. On the European continent, the Spanish used Aloe and carried it to their New World possessions in the Caribbean and South America. And, of course, Aloe is used in the United States and Canada both as a drink and in cosmetic and ointment products.

Today Aloe vera is grown commercially in the Rio Grande Valley of Texas, in California, in Florida, and in specially-designed greenhouses in Oklahoma--to fill the ever-increasing demand for the real thing.

The Aloe vera plant is widely available to modern households where it is kept for the treatment of burns and other injuries.

Although the known benefits of Aloe vera have limited official standing within the modern medical community, they are strongly supported by authoritative and respected medical writers from Dioscorides, a first century Greek physician, to John P. Heggars, Ph.D., a modern burn researcher.

Those who use Aloe vera should heed the words of Dioscorides, who said that the healing properties are found in the yellowish to liver- colored, offensive smelling, bitter- tasting juice.

So-called 100 per cent Aloe vera products available on the market today, most of which do not meet the description of Dioscorides, might be questionable. A simple rule of thumb to follow is if the product you are thinking of buying looks like water, smells like water, and tastes like water, most likely you're not getting pure Aloe vera but are buying mostly water.

Advertising is responsible for creating and perpetuating many myths and misconceptions regarding Aloe vera. While the First Amendment to the Constitution of the United States gives us the right to say almost anything we want, common sense and honesty demands that we accept the responsibility to seek and find the truth before we open our mouths.

Unfortunately, too many people believe that just because something is printed on the page it must be true. Instead of simply accepting what he's told, the consumer would be wise to consider the facts (and the source of the facts) before spending their money for Aloe vera products.

The Webster dictionary defines a miracle as, "an extraordinary event manifesting outstanding or unusual event, thing, or accomplishment; and a divinely natural occurrence that must be learned humanly." If we were to use Webster's as a definitive gauge, is it any wonder Aloe vera is commonly referred to as a miracle plant?

As in all things, the true test of Aloe vera lies within oneself. Is Aloe vera a miracle plant? Facts are available; please, read on and decide for yourself.

CHAPTER THREE

FROM THE DAWN OF MANKIND

It took early man thousands of years of trial and error to determine which plants were safe to eat and which plants or parts of plants could be used as medicine. This hard-earned knowledge was bought with the blood, sweat, and tears of many, both then and now. Such earned knowledge affords valuable answers to many medical problems, but unfortunately, much of this information has been dismissed as myth and magic without investigation.

Certainly ancient medical practices did, and still do, mix medication with religious beliefs and magical rites. But is that a logical reason for the modern scientific community to completely dismiss Aloe vera's value? Or should all those concerned with the health and well being of mankind continue to explore all possibilities and dismiss none without critical evaluation?

Aloe vera, A Journey Through the Ages

One of the earliest, if not the first, book (or "Materia Medica") on the subject of natural medication was the Rig Vede compiled in India between 4500-1600 B.C. This book lists hundreds of plants used for medicine; however, it does not mention the use of Aloe. Some authorities believe that a Twenty-First Century B.C. Sumerian clay tablet, found in the city of Nippur, includes Aloe in its list of useful medical plants. As a matter of fact, the first detailed discussion of Aloe's medical value is found in the "Papyrus Ebers", an Egyptian document, written between 1553-50 B.C. This document gives twelve formulas for the use of Aloe, mixed with other natural agents, to be used as a treatment for a number of internal and external human disorders.

Milestones and Benchmarks

The first milestone in western man's detailed understanding of medical plants is found in the books of Hippocrates (460-375 B.C.) who is often referred to as the father of western medicine, but his Materia Medica makes no mention of Aloe. During that same period, the plant, according to Copra's "Indigenous Drugs of India", had apparently come of age in India, where it was widely used. Copra writes, "The uses of aloes, the common musabbar, for external application on inflamed painful parts of the body and for causing purgation are too well know in India to need any special mention. Its application in medicine dates back to the 4th century B.C."

In Greek pharmacology, the plant was first mentioned by Celsius (25 B.C. 50 A.D.), but his comments are limited to the use of Aloe and its power as a purgative.

The first western benchmark in our understanding of Aloe is the "Greek Herbal" of Dioscorides (41-68 AD.) This master of Roman pharmacy developed his knowledge and skill traveling with the armies of Rome. Dioscorides expands our understanding by giving the first detailed description of the plant we call Aloe vera and notes specifically that it is the bitter juices which drain from the leaf, the sap not the gel, which heals.

He writes that the plant "has a leaf like Squill, thick, fat, somewhat broad in its compass, broken or bowbacked behind, and both sides of the leaf are prickly, appearing thin and short...All of it has a strong scent and is very bitter to the taster...It has the power of binding, of inducing sleep, of drying, of thickening of the body, it loosens the belly, and the cleansing of the stomach by drinking two spoonsful with cold water or warm milk".

He added that this bitter aloe is a treatment for boils and ulcerated genitals, heals the foreskin, is good for dry itchy skin irritation, works on hemorrhoids, takes away bruises, stops the loss of hair, is good for the tonsils, gums and for general mouth pain, and works as eye medicine when roasted in a hot vessel and mixed with water. Dioscordes further states that the whole leaf when pulverized will stop the bleeding of wounds.

Another famous physician of the period, Pliny the Elder (A.D. 23-79), generally repeated the findings of Dioscorides but did add some new details, further enhancing man's understanding of Aloe vera. He claimed that the plant helps check perspiration, and that the root could be boiled down and used as a treatment for leprous sores.

Pliny says that "The kind (of Aloe vera) most approved grows in the regions of Colophon, Mysis a Priene. This is shiny, as like as possible to bull glue, spongy with very fine cracks, quickly melting, with a bad smell." Both Dioscorides and Pliny state that even in the First Century A.D., there were those who would defraud the buyer by making and selling less than the real thing. As Pliny put it, "the bastard scamonium, is made generally in Judaea [sic], with flour of bitter vetch...being like milk to the touch of the tongue, extremely light and turning white when dissolved. The bastard kind being detected by the taste, for the genuine burns the tongue." It is clear from a study of Pliny that he also dried the whole leaf of the Aloe in formulating some of his medicines.

By the end of the Second Century A.D., the plant had become an important part of Western pharmacopoeia used by Galen, Antyllus, Aretacus and some other physicians. It was also used throughout the Middle East, and the trade in Aloe from east to west was extensive. The best Aloe was grown east of the Roman territory.

The next addition to our knowledge of Aloe vera is found in the Chinese Materia Medicas (Seventh Century-Seventeenth Century AD.). Aloe was known by the name of Lu-hui (meaning "black deposit" a reference to its dark color) or Hsiang-tqan (meaning elephant's gall, a reference to its bitter taste). These papers make special note of Aloe's value as a treatment for sinusitis and as a treatment for worm fever and convulsions in children, all by internal administration. The Chinese also re-confirm the plant's use as a treatment for skin afflictions.

From the Ninth Century, we find the writings of Al-Kindi, a philosopher, engineer, and physician of great note in the

Arab world. He mainly repeats earlier information but does add that the Syrians call the Aloe vera plant sabhra or sebara, and that the Arabs call it sabir or sabr, in both cases the meaning is the same--bitter and shining substance. He did, however, indicate its use for inflammatory pain, and related Aloe's effective use for eye ulcers, for dyspnea, and for "melancholy." Further, he notes Aloe's ophthalmological uses. In Al-Kindi's day, Aloe vera was employed in Iran as a well-known purgative, and in Egypt as a detersive, desecrate, and as an emmenagogue.

Over the next 1000 years, we find many, many similar reports by physicians around the world, changing little except for a few variations in the use of Aloe vera.

Even though some of these scholarly papers have helped separate fact from fiction, today most books, brochures, pamphlets, magazine articles, and other writings on the subject of Aloe vera continue to repeat most, if not all, of the historical, medical, and chemical myths about the plant.

MYTHS

In a 1961 article in Economic Botany, Julie F. Morton wrote that processors of Aloe vera, although often "inadequately financed," were "heavily armed with Biblical references (which are entirely inapplicable to the fresh leaf) and with other evidence such as testimonials from lay-persons, laboratories, doctors, hospitals.. .." With this evidence, much of it impressive, the promoters seek to gain official recognition of the virtues of their respective products. Unfortunately for those who produce a quality product, the exploitation of

Aloe preparations has too often been accompanied by misinformation and exaggerated claims, usually in advertising literature and commercially inspired articles in the press and in popular magazines. The public, bombarded with both honest and semi-fictional claims, becomes confused and wary of all Aloe vera products.

One example of this is a persistent myth, traced to the Florida Seminoles, concerning the use of Aloe leaf pulp in surgery. This tale is not borne out by the ethnobotanical studies of Dr. William Sturtevant of the Smithsonian Institution and it is flatly denied by the tribal medicine men interrogated by Mr. Albert DeVane, of Lake Placid, at the request of Morton. Such tales only add to the "patent medicine racket aura and repel many whom the exploiters desire to impress," Morton concludes.

Undoubtedly the most despicable misuse of the name "Aloes" is that which claims the medicine plant is mentioned in the Bible. All annotated reference Bibles state that the Aloes of the Bible are NOT ALOE VERA, but are the perfumed wood (Latin Lignum Aloes) from the East Indian Aloes tree (Aquilaria agallocha). The oil from this wood was used by the Hebrews to perfume their beds, to anoint their bodies, and to cover the odor of decaying flesh during the burial ceremony. The following Bible verses are commonly used by the uninformed to promote Aloe vera products.

Numbers 24:6 --"As the valleys are they spread forth, as gardens by the river's side, as the trees of lign aloes which the Lord hath planted, and as cedar trees beside the water."

Psalms 45:8 --"All thy garments smell of myrrh, and aloes and cassia, out of the ivory places, whereby they had made thee glad."

Proverbs 7:17 --"I have perfumed my bed with myrrh, aloes, and cinnamon".

Song of Solomon 4:14 --"Spikenard and saffron; calamus and cinnamon, with all trees of frankincense; myrrh and aloes, with all the chief spices."

Of all the Biblical references, the ones that are always used by promoters are found in John 19:39 thru 40; however, like the others they are references to the use of a perfume, used in this instance to cover the odor of decaying flesh.

John 19:39 -- "And there came also, Nicodemus, which at the first came Jesus by night, and brought a mixture of myrrh, and aloes, about a hundred pounds weight." And...

John 19:40 -- "Then took they the body of Jesus and wound it in linen cloth with the spices, as the manner of the Jews is to bury."

Despite universal agreement among scholars that the references are to aloes wood, NOT ALOE VERA, this and many other myths continue to surround the plant. For example, it is widely reported that Aristotle convinced Alexander the Great to conquer the island of Socotra in order to obtain an adequate supply of Aloe to heal the wounds of his soldiers. In fact, records of Alexander do not refer to any such conquest. This idea is discredited by the location of Socotra, which is at the eastern end of the Gulf of Aden (an arm of the Indian Ocean between Aden and Somalia), some 1,500 miles south of the southernmost point of Alexander's conquests.

Another wonderful story which is, nevertheless, untrue is the one that Nefertiti and Cleopatra credited Aloe vera gel for their legendary beauty. Supporters of this idea state that the plant is depicted on many Egyptian tombs and temple walls in both drawings and paintings. Other proponents of this claim go so far as to say that the paintings show servants bringing forth vessels of fresh Aloe vera gel and handing them to Cleopatra. Numerous researchers have concluded that no such drawings exist.

Others have used the good name of Marco Polo, stating that he found the Chinese using Aloe vera as a treatment for rashes and other skin disorders and for stomach ailments. While it is true that during the time of Marco Polo's visit, the Chinese mixed Aloe with licorice and used it as a wash for eczematous skin affections, (as outlined in the Chinese Materia Medica Vegetable Kingdom, released simultaneously in Peking and Shanghai in the 1920's and 1930's), Marco Polo does not mention Aloe vera, although he does mention aloes wood.

Another famous explorer, Christopher Columbus is also erroneously linked with Aloe vera in two versions of a distorted tale. The first states that Columbus carried potted Aloe vera plants on his first voyage to the new world as a treatment for sunburn, cuts, scrapes, abrasions, and other shipboard injuries. The second claims that the explorer found Aloe vera growing on the islands of the new world and brought them on board his ships for the same purpose.

Both stories have their origins in the fact that Columbus mentions aloes in his log of October 21, 1492, and again on October 23, 1492. He wrote, "I see thousands of sorts of trees...and thousands of sorts of plants...and of the whole lot I only recognize Aloes much of which I ordered aboard." The only problem with this story is that there are no species of

Aloe vera native to North America. Therefore we know that Columbus mistook the Agave (Century Plant) for Aloe vera, the Agave being similar in appearance, having spear-shaped leaves, but it is not American Aloe (vera)--a mistake which is still made today.

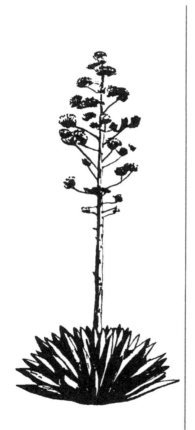

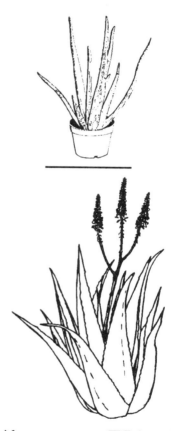

Agave (Century Plant)-- Not American Aloe (vera).

Aloe vera pup (T.R.) and a mature Aloe vera Linne (A. Barbadensis Miller) (B.R.).

PART II

MAGIC

CHAPTER FOUR

THE MAGIC OF BELIEVING

Today, scientists, who realize that the cure for man's ills are not always found in a sterile test tube, are listening to folk tales around the world. Clawing their way through the jungles, they seek to talk with tribal medicine men who use incantations, spells, and magic in addition to plant-derived medications to achieve healing. The scientists are gathering samples of plants used by these practitioners for chemical evaluation in an attempt to discover if the plants contain natural healing chemicals.

This search is not a new phenomenon but has been going on as long as men have sought wisdom and knowledge. These scientists do not dismiss any possibility but seek truth wherever it can be found.

Since World War II, medical science has, for the most part, dismissed folk medicine as the ravings of misguided purveyors of magic, yet today many of the drugs available from the drug store contain plants or plant extracts (or, in some cases, synthetic versions of the real thing). Some examples include digitalis (foxglove), astringents and antiseptics (golden seal), laxative agents (rhubarb, senna root, and Aloe), aspirin (derived from the bark of the wintergreen and sweet birch tree), and Valium (valerine root).

In October, 1987, Dr. Mark Plotkin, appearing on Nova, a nationally televised program of the Public Broadcasting Service, said that in 1974 the United States imported medicinal plants costing more than twenty four million dollars, and then turned them into medicines which sold for more than three billion dollars. It is a fairly significant business.

During the early years of the twentieth century, pharmaceutical companies studied thousands of plants. From those plants they derived many of the agents which are mentioned above. However, since the 1950's this method has been mostly abandoned due to the fact that it is much cheaper to find and produce the agents synthetically than to find and extract them from plants. Major drug manufacturing companies also realize that natural agents cannot be patented and therefore cannot be controlled. This is especially true for a plant like Aloe vera, which is already in widespread use by the public.

As a matter of economics, the decision of the pharmaceutical houses makes perfect sense. This is probably the major reason that pharmaceutical houses have not pursued the truth about Aloe vera, relegating that responsibility to promoters in the health food and cosmetic industries. Unfortunately, many of these promoters play fast and loose with the truth, putting economic gain above the health and well-being of humanity.

Some of the promoters say, and maybe even believe, that they hold the secret to some magic process or formula which makes their Aloe vera juice unique and superior to all others. This belief may be justified if their juice is properly processed and stabilized (preserved in its natural state), if their plants are grown under the best possible conditions, and if their product contains an adequate amount of Aloe vera juice (including the sap). And the questions remain -- is it the plant, is it the processing; or is it both? While there are secrets that remain to be discovered, the keys to Aloe vera's efficacy lie in its chemistry, not in a tapestry of tales.

However, before totally dismissing the value of "magic" it might be useful to look at the folk uses of the plant and compare them to the scientific facts.

CHAPTER FIVE

FOLKLORE AROUND THE WORLD

Used in the East as a charm, Aloe vera was hung over the door to keep out evil spirits and was worn around the neck as an amulet to insure a happy, healthy life. Some may laugh at such ideas and use them to justify their conclusion that Aloe vera be relegated to the realm of superstition. Don't laugh too hard, for our ancestors may have known many secrets we fail to see.

In Colombia, for instance, children's legs and feet are coated with the ground-up plant as protection from insect bites. Research has shown that the Aloe vera has value as an insect repellent because of its bitter taste and the odor of the sap, probably the reasons insects don't bother a healthy plant.

In African folklore, we find that hunters anointed themselves with the juice of the plant. The user probably believed it to be beneficial to a successful hunt. Actually the foul odor of the Aloe vera juice may have covered the body odor of the hunter or blocked perspiration, making it harder for animals to smell the hunter.

According to other African folk tales, many tribes required everybody in the village to bathe publicly in an infusion of Aloe in case of an epidemic of colds. This, too, may not be such a strange idea, for modern studies have repeatedly shown that Aloe vera is an effective germ-killer in both internal and external use.

The people of many ancient civilizations anointed themselves with the juice of the plant mixed with perfumes and oils as a part of religious or ceremonial rites. What may have started as a simple religious act perhaps led them to discover that Aloe, when rubbed on the forehead and temples, could help "heal the head" or alleviate headaches. Such an effect is described by Dioscorides and in the Papyrus Ebers. Indeed, if one considers that scientific studies have shown that Aloe is a vaso-dilator (opens the blood vessels) and that some headaches (migraine) are due to blood vessel restriction, then it would be only fair to conclude that the ancients weren't so stupid after all.

The Egyptians, and many other early peoples, believed that plants had magic power and assigned them royal status within their household. This may have led to the legend that the Egyptians kept Aloe as a palace plant, assigning it status second only to the pharaoh, the royal family, and certain animals. This legend about Aloe vera may be true. Remember the Papyrus Ebers already mentioned.

It is almost certain that either Spanish Jesuits or African slaves brought Aloe to the New World, probably to the island of Barbados, in about 1590. Spanish missionaries in the Western Hemisphere always planted Aloe around their settlements and carried it on their journeys to aid the sick. Legend has it that the Indians of both Central America and Mexico learned to use Aloe for treatment of burns, skin and stomach ulcerations, intestinal disorders, kidney disorders, and an enhancement of longevity and sexual powers. To the Indian the plant must have seemed a wonder from the Gods--carried around, as it was, by powerful religious men. They called it, simply, "Wands of Heaven" (a reference both to the shape of leaves and the fact that they seemed to point toward Heaven).

In China, special herbal blends, including Aloe vera, were believed to possess magical properties capable of producing desirable results--good health, happiness, wealth, love, friendship, longevity and sexual prowess. The Chinese mixed Aloe vera with licorice and drank it as a tonic. Their reports seem to indicate that the tonic made them "feel better." Although the condition of "feeling better" may seem vague, it may be linked to Aloe's ability to detoxify the body, a phenomenon reported by Dr. Jeffrey Bland, Linus Pauling Institute, in his medical paper, "Effect of Orally Consumed Aloe vera Juice on Gastrointestinal Function In Normal Humans," published in 1985 and discussed in detail in this book under the chapter "Toxicology". One can conclude that perhaps the Chinese achieved an effective combination of herb and faith which was less magic and more folkloric medicine.

As demonstrated here, the key to many of the secrets of Aloe vera is readily available to those who seek the truth through investigation. We can gain access to many ancient secrets that hold valuable information, and although old ideas have been misused, that does not mean that they do not hold valuable information.

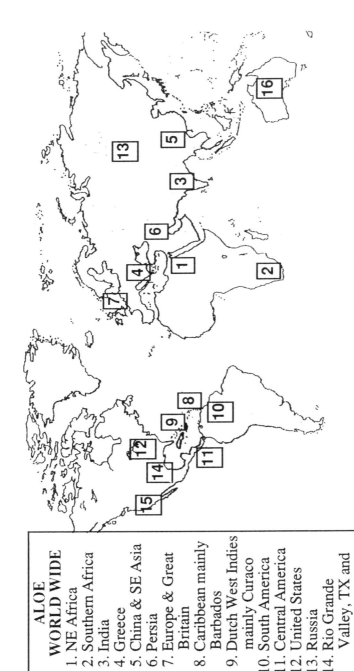

ALOE
WORLD WIDE
1. NE Africa
2. Southern Africa
3. India
4. Greece
5. China & SE Asia
6. Persia
7. Europe & Great
   Britain
8. Caribbean mainly
   Barbados
9. Dutch West Indies
   mainly Curaco
10. South America
11. Central America
12. United States
13. Russia
14. Rio Grande
    Valley, TX and
    Oklahoma
15. California
16. Australia

Refrences 1 and 2 show the origin of Aloe vera. Refrences 3 thru 16 represent the chronological order of how Aloe vera has been transplanted world-wide during the last 3,500 years.

PART III

MEDICINE

CHAPTER SIX

GEL, SAP, OR WHOLE LEAF?

The most wide-spread myth accepted by today's consumer of Aloe vera products is that it was the nearly tasteless and colorless center of the plant, commonly known as the gel, that was used in antiquity as the healing agent. As a matter of fact, all ancient documents on the subject point directly to the bitter, yellowish (or reddish) sap of the plant as the medicinal agent. The documents also show that the whole leaf was often ground up and used as a poultice or was eaten as a treatment for many internal disorders.

Modern medical and scientific reports cause further confusion by using the words "gel," "Aloe vera gel or jelly," or simply "Aloe gel or jelly" in their texts, making it unclear what part of the plant the scientists are actually experimenting with; however, details within these texts repeatedly show that the sap was present in the Aloe vera product used in all successful studies.

This fact is clearly demonstrated by the statements of C. E. Collins, D.D.S., M.D., and Creston Collins, M.S., who said in their March, 1935 paper "Roentgen Dermatitis Treated With Fresh Whole Leaf of Aloe Vera" published in the <u>American Journal of</u> <u>Roentgenology and Radium Therapy,</u>

"the substance used was scraped from the center of the leaf, and had a yellow color similar to lemon Jello [sic]." This statement shows that the product used was a combination of the sap and the gel because the sap is the only part of the plant which has a "yellow" color.

Additional clarification of this fact was added in 1938 by Archie Fine, M.D. and Samuel Brown, M.D. of The Tumor Clinic and the Department of Roetgenology, respectively, Jewish Hospital in Cincinnati, Ohio, "The flat outer covering is trimmed away with a sharp knife, exposing the transparent GREENISH-YELLOW pulp which is crisscrossed by several knife cuts so as to cause the leaf to bleed..." and "Another method is to scrape the jelly from the leaf, apply it to the lesion and keep it in place with wax paper or oiled silk dressing until it dries out or is absorbed." These statements clearly show that both teams were preparing the Aloe leaves in a manner which caused large amounts of yellowish sap to be included with the colorless gel.

In August, 1939, Dr. J. E. Crewe, M.D., a practicing physician in Rochester, Minnesota, published, "Aloe In The Treatment of Burns and Scalds," which describes the use of two ointments prepared from Aloe vera. One was made from Socotrine aloes which are dark brown; the other was made from Barbados aloes, a product which is almost black. Crewe's statements indicate that the ointments prepared by him were mostly sap.

In 1941, Thomas D. Rowe, Professor of Pharmacy at the University of Virginia Medical School, in his paper, "Further Observations On The Use of Aloe Vera Leaf in the Treatment of Third Degree X-Ray Reactions," said that experimental use of the plant led him to the conclusion that the healing agent was in the rind (where the sap is found). Although Rowe's studies are important, they have created a great deal of confusion, for while some of Rowe's experiments were highly successful, others were utter failures. Actually, the failures demonstrate that it is the sap that healed, for the Rowe report states that two explanations were possible for the failure. The first failure Rowe attributed to the poor condition of some of the leaves. He says that, "Most of the juice, or latex, had drained from the leaves during shipment and it is probable that the healing agent was lost in this way." A second suggestion was provided by the grower of the Aloe leaves used in the experiment. The grower said that the healing agent "may not be present in the leaves at all times, but is found there only during certain seasons of the year." This is an idea which was first noted by Pliny the Elder, some 1,900 years earlier. The obvious conclusion is that if the sap is not present, the product will not heal.

R. Y. Gottschall, in his "Antibacterial Substances In Seed Plants Active Against Tubercle Bacilli," a 1950 medical paper published in the <u>American Review of Tuberculosis</u> (with colleagues J. C. Jennings, L. E. Weller, C. T. Redemann, E. H. Lucas, and H. M. Sell), pointed directly to the sap as the healing agent, when he said that the antimicrobial effects of Aloe vera were confined to its "Barbaloin" or sap. In 1953, C. C. Lushbaugh, M.D., and D. B. Hale, B.S., in the paper, "Experimental Acute Radiodermatitis Following Beta Irradiation--V. Histopathological Study of the Mode of Action of Therapy with Aloe vera," indicated that in their experimental procedures, the fresh whole leaf of the Aloe vera plant was used. According to the scientists, "the fresh leaf was applied by removing the rind from the flat side of a 2 x 1 inch piece of leaf and placing the exposed inner jelly-like substance in contact with the irradiated area. The rind on the outside of the piece aided in holding the jelly in place because it provided a stiff surface to which adhesive tape could adhere." Thus, they made it perfectly clear that the sap was present because the rind was left in place.

The importance of the sap as the active healing agent in Aloe vera was further substantiated by Julian J. Blitz, D.O., James W. Smith, D.O., and Jack H. Gerard, D.O., South Memorial Hospital and Clinic, Dania, Florida, in their paper published in 1962 in the Journal of the American Osteopathic Association. They wrote that "the substance used was slightly acrid and possessed a somewhat disagreeable odor." This description makes it clear that the sap was present, even though the authors titled their report, "Aloe vera gel in peptic ulcer therapy: Preliminary report." In this instance, the presence of sap can be deduced from the description given, for the clear part of the plant (the gel) has no odor; only the sap is characteristically "acrid" having a "somewhat disagreeable odor."

Two more recent studies show the importance of the sap. A 1964 paper, "Bacteriostatic Property of Aloe vera" by microbiologists Lorna J. Lorenzetti, Rupert Salisbury, Jack L. Beal, and Jack N. Baldwin, which was published in the Journal of Pharmaceutical Sciences, describes the preparation of the Aloe used. "Leaves of Aloe vera Linne were cut at the base and stood upright so that the juice could drain from the leaves into receptacles." This makes it clear that the subject of this study is the sap, because the sap is the only part of the leaf which will drain in such a manner. And, "While the freeze-dried whole leaf minus the juice, the leaf mesophyll, and the leaf epidermis of Aloe vera Linne did not exhibit bacteriostatic properties, the freeze-dried juice previously heated for 15 minutes at 80 degrees did inhibit S. aureus 209, S. pyogenes, C. xerose, and S. paralypin using the agar diffusion test method." This study reconfirms the findings of Gottschall (1949) that it is the sap that contains the plant's antibacterial agents.

Lastly, in the 1973 paper, "Use of Aloe in Treating Leg Ulcers and Dermatoses," M. El Zawahry, M.D., M. Rashad Hegazy, M.D., and M. Helal, B.Ph., Ph.Ch. of the medical faculty of Cairo University wrote, "the fresh leaves were cut, transversely from the base and left for 48 hours so that the bitter substance would drain off. The leaves were opened and the gel was extracted from the leaf. It was homogenized and filtered through muslin, a preservative was added and it was stored under refrigeration." As is obvious from this quote, the researchers believed that by simply cutting the leaf and draining it, all the sap would be eliminated. However, this assumption is erroneous, as is shown by the chemical analysis of the product after preparation [which is given in the report]. The report states that the product used contained steroids and chlorides which are components of the sap and not of the gel.

Fresh or Processed?

Reports of the condition of Aloe leaves used in experiments during the 1930's and 1940's cast great doubt on another aspect of the modern propaganda of some Aloe promoters--which is that the leaf must be fresh to be effective. Several reports of successful experiments make it clear that the leaf used was not fresh and that the term "fresh" was used to denote "not spoiled." Indeed, after the leaves were cut from the plant, they were shipped over long distances--a fact which is apparent from the reports of Colonel H. W. Johnston, who started growing Aloe vera in Florida in 1912. According to Julie Morton who interviewed Johnston, Johnston reported that he shipped leaves to various pharmaceutical concerns after drying them in his attic. He also sold "fresh" leaves in the local marketplace for treatment of skin afflictions, for arthritic joints, for use as a mild laxative, and for stomach ulcers. He said that for the latter purpose, the pulp was generally diced, placed in a jar of water, and refrigerated. Collins and Collins indicated that the leaves used in experiments were cut from plants grown in the Florida Everglades. That the leaves used were not freshly cut is indicated by a statement by Fine and Brown, "Leaves keep fairly well if covered with wax paper and kept in a cool atmosphere, not below 50 or above 70 degrees." But the most telling remark was made by Rowe when he stated that the Aloe leaf did not need to be fresh to be effective.

Even more dramatic is Rowe's statement that the leaf was still effective after it appeared to be rotten. This was further confirmed by Gottschall, who made it perfectly clear that the product still worked, even after processing. From these reports it is obvious that the leaf does not have to be freshly cut to be effective; it is also apparent that if the sap is not present, the product does not work.

Processing and use -- old and new

Historical records contain useful information on the best way to select and process the Aloe vera plant to obtain the healing agent. The ancients removed the leaf from the plant, cut off the butt (fat end) and collected the sap into a pot or animal skin; or they left the leaf on the plant, made a small slit at the base of the leaf and allowed the sap to drip on the ground, on an animal skin, or in a pot. The sap was then boiled or dried in the sun and packed in earthen vessels or animal skins for shipment.

Dioscorides was the first to fully explain how to select and use this processed Aloe. He said, "There are two kinds of the juice, one which is sandy and seems to be the purest, the other like liver. Choose the one that is pure, unadulterated and unstoney, glittering, yellowish, brittle, liver-like, easily melted and excelling in bitterness. Refuse the one that is black and hard to break. They [the processors] dilute it with gum, which parallels Aloe's taste, bitterness and odor and does not fall apart even in the slightest when it is squeezed between the fingers." Dioscorides states that Aloe should always be mixed with other natural agents, including water and milk, when taken internally. He added that it can be mixed with other purgative medicines, to make them milder and "less harmful to the stomach". When used externally, Aloe was recommended to be mixed with Rosin, sod honey, sweet wine, honey, acetum and Rosaceum. For severe infections, such as "wounds and... boils," Dioscorides recommended that the sap be dried to a powder and sprinkled directly on the area to be treated.

Dioscorides observed that the sap will not flow freely from plants grown under less than ideal conditions. Dioscorides said that the best Aloe comes from India, but also noted that "it also grows in Arabia and Asia and in certain sea-bordering places and islands, as in Andros, the plants from here are not good for extracting juice but are fit for the stopping of bleeding or wounds when pulverized and applied directly." In other words, Indian Aloe appeared to be the best because the growing conditions were better than in other locations.

Pliny the Elder, repeated most of Dioscorides but added that Aloe can be mixed with rue boiled in rose oil to check perspiration. Pliny said, "Near the rising of the Dog Star (in the spring before the plant flowers) a hollow is made in this root, so that the juice may collect in it automatically; this is dried in the sun and worked into lozenges...Some (time) before the seed ripens, make an incision in the stem (actually just above the stem at the base of the leaves) to get the juice; some do so to the leaves as well." Pliny further describes the product of choice, "So the best aloes will be fatty and shiny, of a ruby color, friable, compact like liver, and easily melted. Pliny adding, "The nature of an aloe is bracing, astringent, and gently warming."

The ancient manuscripts contain instructions on the correct method of processing Aloe for human use. They indicate that Aloe was almost always heated whether by drying in the sun, boiling in a pot, or roasting in a pan--it seems to have made no difference. So apparently the ancients knew that heating does not destroy the active healing ingredients of Aloe vera.

Hot or Cold?

In spite of scientific proof to the contrary, the false idea that heating destroys Aloe vera's active ingredients, and therefore its ability to heal, continues to be perpetrated by those who claim that their product is "cold processed."

The earliest modern study which points out that Aloe's healing ingredients are not destroyed by heat is the 1933 report "Tissue Therapy in Cutaneous Leishmaniasis" by V. P. Filatov, a Russian. This study was first published in the United States in the American Review of Soviet Medicine in August, 1945. In his report Filatov says he heated and sterilized Aloe at not more than 70 degrees centigrade for an hour daily. He says he repeats this process each day for three days, allowing the product to cool at room temperature between heatings.

In 1949, R. Y. Gottschall did the first well-controlled study of the germ-killing power of Aloe (by which Gottschall meant the sap alone), when he examined 161 species of seed-plants. The extracts of 27 were found to have anti-bacterial activity against Mycobacterium tuberculosis. Of these plants, he found two to have superior killing effects on this bacillus, and the best of all was Aloe vera Linne (A. chineusis Baker).

Another medical paper by Gottshall, "Antibacterial Substances in Seed Plants Active Against Tubercle Bacilli," published in the American Review of Tuberculosis, reconfirmed the fact that it is the barbaloin which is responsible for the anti-microbial activity of Aloe vera and related specific detail concerning how the product was processed. The researchers state that, "All of the extracts were stabilized by heating at 121 degrees Centigrade for fifteen minutes before being assayed since the active principles from both A. vera and M. canadense were heat stable." In other words, heat does not destroy the anti- microbial agents in Aloe, and it is necessary to heat the product to produce stability.

In 1964, in the Journal of Pharmaceutical Sciences, Lorna J. Lorenzetti, Rupert Salisbury, Jack L. Beal, and Jack N. Baldwin, in their paper " Bacteriostatic Property of Aloe vera," said, "Leaves of A. vera L. (Aloe vera Linne) were cut at the base and stood upright so that the juice could drain from the leaves into receptacles. If tested immediately, the fresh juice exhibited a marked zone of inhibition of S. aureus 209. However, the principle responsible for the inhibitory activity was found to be unstable.

Preservatives such sodium bisulfite, sodium benzoate, and methyl paraben were ineffective; however, the principle could be temporarily preserved by refrigeration and preserved for an even longer period by heating the juice for 15 minutes at 80 degrees." Note: 80 degrees centigrade. This study also agrees with Gottschall's opinion that sap is the source of the anti-microbial agents.

The report goes on to add that Aloe not only is active against Mycobacterium tuberculosis (Gottschall) but concludes that it is a broad spectrum germ controlling agent effective against E. coli, Strep tococcus pyrogenes, Corymebacterium xerose, Singelia paradysenlarias, salmanella typhosa, Salmonella scholturuellera, and Sclreonella paratypns."

The scientists concluded that the anti-microbial agents are

in the sap. "While the freeze-dried whole leaf minus the juice of the leaf mesophyll and the leaf epidermis of A. vera L. did not exhibit bacteriostatic properties; the freeze-dried juice previously heated for 15 minutes at 80 degrees did inhibit S. aureus 209, S. pyogenes, C. zerose, and S partypin using the agar diffusion method" This statement leaves no doubt that the researchers found that the rind of the plant or the mucilage is not responsible for the plant's anti- bacterial capabilities.

In 1975, a short communication concerning the brandykininase (anti-inflammatory) activity of Aloe extract was published by the Institute of Pharmacaognosy, Fujita-Gakuen University, Hisai, Mie, Japan. The principal authors are Keisuke Fujita, Ryoji Teradaira and Toshiharu Nagatsu, Department of Biochemistry, School of Dentistry, Aichi-Gakuin University, Nagoya, Japan. In this study, the researchers used an extract of the fresh leaves of Aloe and filtered it through an extra-fine membrane to capture all components with a molecular weight higher than 10,000. The material was then dissolved in water to make a concentration of 30 milligrams of powder per milliliter. Before heating this product, the researchers ran a brandykininase activity test which showed little activity. They then boiled the extract and repeated the test. The heated extracts showed much greater brandykininase activity than the one processed at room temperature. This test supports the theory that Aloe has outstanding anti-inflammatory capacity, and that this capability is not destroyed by heat, but is, in fact, greatly enhanced by heating.

All of the preceeding reports, both ancient and modern, not only confirm the theory that Aloe's anti-microbial agents are in the sap, they also confirm that the anti-inflammatory and other active principals (healing aspects) of the plant are in Aloe (sap), and that heating does not destroy these principles, but, in fact, enhances them.

Ask yourself the following questions: Is there any information in antiquity to support the idea that the gel alone was used as a healing agent or was it the sap that was used? Are there any modern studies which demonstrate that the gel alone has ever been used successfully to heal, or was the sap present in all successful studies? Does scientific evidence support the idea that heating Aloe vera destroys its healing principals, or does the evidence show exactly the opposite. Does the evidence indicate that Aloe vera can or should be "cold processed"? And what does "cold processed" mean, anyway?

Every scientific report and bit of historical evidence this author has seen makes it absolutely clear that the healing agents of Aloe are found only in the sap, not in the gel, and that heating does not destroy these principals but does, in fact, enhance them.

Please, at this point, do not assume that we are discounting the value of the gel, for I will assure you that we are not. It is important in the overall understanding of how Aloe vera works to heal, and even though the sap alone heals, the presence of the gel in a finished product is important. This is a fact that will become very apparent as we discuss the chemistry of the whole leaf.

If the facts presented thus far are not convincing, we suggest you obtain a plant (or leaf) and process it yourself. Here's how. With leaf in hand, cut off the bottom of the leaf and look closely at the severed end to make sure that the yellow sap is present. The sap will drip from the tubes between the green outer rind and the mucous-like gel. If the leaf contains only a small amount of sap, it can still be seen but will not drip or run from the leaf. You can test for the presence of the sap by rubbing your finger over the severed end and tasting the juice to detect whether it is bitter or not. If the juice is not bitter, then the leaf either does not contain the sap because of seasonal depletion, or like Columbus, you may even have the wrong plant.

Split the leaf lengthwise and scrape out all of the center portion down to the rind. Pulverize the material in a blender or food processor and boil it in a glass or stainless steel pan for at least five minutes. Notice the color. Notice the odor. Notice the mess. Notice that the thick mucilage turns to a water-like liquid. And, if you're an Aloe vera drinker, notice the taste. If you have a cut, scrape, injury, insect bite, burn or other discomfort rub a little of your product on it and notice the beneficial effects and decide for yourself.

If you have product left over, refrigerate or freeze it and use as needed. If refrigerated, the product should last from two to three weeks, and if frozen, for several months. Neither heating nor freezing destroys the beneficial effects of Aloe, and it need not be "fresh" to be effective. At this point if you are not too tired--stand up, raise your right hand in the air, turn your palm around and pat yourself on the back, for you are now an official Aloe vera processor. Like any Aloe vera processor worth his salt, you know that Aloe vera must be heated to preserve it and that heating does not destroy its beneficial effects. You also understand the importance of the combination of sap and the gel and that even when the gel is used alone, it must be heated to destroy the organisms which contaminate the product during processing.

By now it should be evident that the gel is not responsible for healing, that the healing agents are in the sap, and that heat does not destroy them.

Today, the patent medicine racket Morton described thirty years ago is still very much a part of the Aloe vera industry. All too many within the Aloe vera industry promote the myth and magic, not the medicine, of Aloe despite the fact that the medical and scientific evidence is available. The quick-buck artists and pseudo-experts have promoted Aloe products (most of which contain little or no Aloe) because there is money to be made by fooling the public.

CHAPTER SEVEN

VEGETABLE JUICE OR MEDICAL MARVEL?

Aloe vera juice, with or without the sap, is classified by the Food and Drug Administration (FDA) as a vegetable juice (food) provided that the juice does not contain more then 50 ppm (parts per million) of the aloin, that it is produced using proper manufacturing practices and meets all of the standards set by regulation of food processing, and that the juice has been stabilized with preservatives and/or food additives which are generally recognized as safe [GRAS] and approved for this propose by FDA.

The Overselling of Aloe vera

Annabel Hecht's article, "The Overselling of Aloe Vera," published in the July/August, 1981, issue of FDA Consumer, defines Aloe vera as, "A common houseplant that has a long and exotic history. In recent years, the plant and its juices have become big business in the do-it-yourself health field, as promoters around the country are selling Aloe vera products with implied claims that their products can cure or alleviate a variety of human complaints."

The article written by Hecht, a member of FDA's public-affairs staff, continues, "FDA is reviewing Aloe, aloin (a derivative), and Aloe vera gel as active ingredients in over-the-counter drugs as part of its massive review of the safety and effectiveness and appropriate labeling of all OTC drugs. Two expert advisory panels have found there is not enough scientific evidence to show that Aloe vera is useful for the treatment of minor burns, cuts and abrasions or for the treatment of minor vaginal irritations. Both panels have recommended that further tests be made before Aloe vera is declared safe and effective for its intended use.

Yet another expert panel has studied the pharmaceutical Aloe and recommended that it be allowed in laxatives, but cautioned that it be used sparingly and not by children under 6 years of age.

FDA has not yet decided whether to accept the panel's recommendations. Until a decision is made and final monographs setting forth the acceptable ingredients and labeling for these classes of OTC drugs are published, drug products containing aloe vera can continue to be sold.

It is interesting to note that, despite the laxative panel's recommendation, a number of medical sources, including the American Medical Association and the American Pharmaceutical Association, say that Aloe vera should not be used in laxatives because it is unpredictable and sometimes violent. It can cause intestinal gripping, cramping, and colic and can affect smooth muscles such as the uterus, making it a dangerous drink for a pregnant woman. Veterinary use of Aloe as a purgative for horses is no longer recommended for the same reason.

Aloe vera in cosmetics comes under a different set of rules. FDA does not have the authority to require that manufacturers test cosmetic products for safety before they go on the market. However, the Agency can take action against a product that proves to be adulterated or misbranded. So far, no problems have been encountered with cosmetics containing Aloe vera.

Exaggerated medical claims notwithstanding, consumers have asked whether there is any real harm in taking Aloe vera as a tonic, one of the suggested uses for the plant. A 1974 study did show that oral doses were not toxic to rats. However, no scientific studies have been done to determine whether drinking aloe vera might be harmful to humans. This is something that should be kept in mind by anyone planning on quaffing a daily dose. In addition, there is the possibility that continued use of an Aloe vera tonic could make a person sensitive to the plant. In that case, later applications of creams or lotions containing Aloe vera might result in an allergic reaction.

Far more serious, however, is the harm that comes when proper medical treatment of serious illness is neglected or abandoned in favor of products that have no proven value. Victims of arthritis and other diseases for which there is no known cure often are easily persuaded to try almost anything in the hope of relief. They, in particular, should be skeptical of any product that is promoted as a cure-all based on testimonials rather than solid scientific evidence."

In 1983 after reading "The Over-selling of Aloe Vera," this writer sent a letter requesting the documentation that FDA reviewed in coming to the conclusion that Aloe vera has little or no proven medical value. Following that request, I received a large body of information from FDA that included many of the modern studies reviewed in this book. Among the studies was the 1974 toxicity study on rats referred to in "The Overselling of Aloe Vera," plus several other toxicity studies which concur with the 1974 study.

Pharmaceutical Aloe, as referred to in the above quote, means "the sap of various species of the plant which has been dried to a powder." This product is yellowish or reddish in color, depending on species, and is extremely bitter to the taste due to its' high concentration. Pharmaceutical Aloe has been officially recognized since the inception of the U.S.P. (United States Pharmacopia) in 1820. Originally the U.S.P. listed six official species from which the sap can be extracted. They are Aloe perryi Baker, Aloe vera Linne, Aloe barbadensis Miller, Aloe spicata Baker, Aloe ferox Lamarck, and Aloe africana Miller. At various times these plants and some others, have been listed as "official" in major pharmacopias worldwide including the British Pharmacopia (B.P.). Today, the U.S.P. recognizes Aloe perryi Baker and Aloe vera Linne as official while Aloe ferox Miller is not official, and the B.P. officially recognizes these three plus Zanzibar Aloe. According to the B. P. , Zanzibar Aloe is from the islands of Socotria and Curacao and from Southern Africa and is a recognized species.

As used here, " official" means that laxatives can be made from the sap of these species only. Laxative products can contain the pure sap or can be made from an extract of the sap which is generally called Aloin. We know according to chemical analyses as listed in U.S. Pharmacopia, that the sap from Aloe perryi Baker contains between 7.5 per cent to 10 per cent Aloin. The sap from Aloe vera Linne contains 18 to 25 per cent Aloin, and the sap from Aloe africana Miller contains 4.5 to 9 per cent Aloin. In complete disregard for the proceeding facts, most promoters of Aloe vera have erroneously stated that the sap IS aloin, when in fact, aloin is only one of many components of the sap. Interestingly enough, the gel alone has no official standing in any pharmacopia anywhere in the world because it contains no known agents recognized as being of any medical value (drugs).

Strange as it seems, however, pharmaceutical Aloe is listed on the U.S. Dispensary as a "topical protectant," but all efforts to determine just what "topical protectant" means (protect the skin?) has proven futile.

The article states, that if pharmaceutical Aloe or aloin is used incorrectly (in too high a dosage over too short a period) it may cause gripping, cramping and colic, and may affect smooth muscles such as the uterus. However, do not be confused. Real Aloe vera juice, beverages, and tonics that are being sold today bear no resemblance to pharmaceutical Aloe, even if they contain legal amounts of the sap which cause them to be yellow in color, and to have a somewhat bitter taste. The amount of sap these products contain is very minute. In other words, what is legally available in today's marketplace is a tonic or drink that is manufactured almost entirely from gel with a trace amount of the sap.

Aloe products must be processed to eliminate contaminants such as mold, bacteria, fungus, and yeast. FDA-approved preservatives are added to control the re-growth of these organisms. Additionally, anti-oxidants are added to protect its color and taste. This is, in fact, what the word "stabilized" means.

Such products will cause none of the problems noted by

the American Medical Association or the American Pharmaceutical Association such as gripping or cramping. The tonic and drink products do not contain enough sap to produce the problems noted unless enormous amounts of them are consumed daily (amounts that are much higher than would normally be recommended).

Ms. Hecht's statement that no daily dosage of Aloe has ever been qualified is misleading. If the writer is referring to the sap, her information is incorrect, for the sap has been used as a laxative for at least 3,500 years and has been studied extensively for that purpose. Most sources state that the recommended dosage of this product to relieve constipation is two to three grains, depending on the species from which the Aloe is obtained.

It is also important to note that it is against common medical practice for physicians to recommend stimulant laxatives such as Aloe, Senna root, Rhubarb root, etc., for pregnant women. So, even though the article may leave the false impression that Aloe used as a laxative ingredient affects the smooth muscles in an unusual way,it is simply not true when it is compared to other stimulant laxatives. It is apparently common knowledge among physicians and pharmacists that stimulant laxatives should not be used during pregnancy. As a matter of fact, such laxatives commonly carry label warnings indicating they should not be used by pregnant women. Perhaps this is the reason that the laxative panel made no special comment concerning the fact that pharmaceutical Aloe either in pure form or in laxative products should not be used by pregnant women.. Furthermore, the FDA article notwithstanding, it appears that no specific study has been conducted to determine whether or not drinking Aloe vera tonic can cause allergic reactions in humans or make them sensitive to the plant or to creams or lotions containing Aloe vera.

Indeed, there is no evidence in either historical documents or scientific studies that the use of the sap or a combination of sap and gel causes allergic reactions. To the contrary, Aloe has been noted repeatedly as a treatment for rashes, topical allergic reactions, and skin disorders. Some note has also been made of its benefits for treatment of nasal and bronchial allergies. The facts would seem to lead any researcher to the conclusion that Aloe causes little or no allergic response, and has been shown to be an effective treatment for such problems.

It is always a serious matter to abandon professional medical care and advice in favor of unproven medical therapy. But, it seems that those who abandon modern medicine most often do so because modern medicine has failed to provide answers. Reason suggests that those on both sides of this debate should wake-up to the fact that neither side has all of the answers to our medical problem or our long-term health and well-being.

Standards

Many of the papers which were used by FDA to "find" that Aloe vera has very little, if any useful purpose have also been used by promoters to create consumer interest in the plant and products made from it. Unfortunately many of the same promoters have led many consumers into buying products which contain little or no Aloe vera--a fact which can be and has been proven by chemical analyses of the products. Although such tests are readily available and are relatively inexpensive, they are not commonly performed by promoters of Aloe vera products (or at least such promoters make little or no mention of any such tests in their promotional material). The consumer can hardly be expected to test the products they buy.

As long as promoters continue to sell colorless, tasteless, odorless, and therefore medically useless, products, the need for standardized testing is imperative. Otherwise, the consumer will continue to believe that just because the label says that the product "contains 100% Aloe vera," "is made with 100% Aloe vera," "is derived from 100% Aloe vera," or "includes 100% Aloe vera," that the product is, in fact, 100% Aloe vera or is pure Aloe vera. Equally misleading are promoter statements that his product is better than anybody else's because it contains Aloe which is stabilized better, preserved better, or some other unsupported statement. Unfortunately, as of this writing, no standard has been established by any governmental or regulatory agency which can guarantee the consumer that the products they are buying even contain Aloe vera, much less how much it contains. Likewise, no regulation insures that claims made by promoters are scientifically correct as to the concentration, quality, or stabilization procedure of Aloe products.

The questions of standards and methods of stabilizing Aloe vera juice and gel were addressed in 1981 by an organization of more than forty Aloe vera growers, processors, and manufacturers of cosmetics and health foods which contain

Aloe vera. This group, known as the National Aloe Science Council (NASC), states in the bylaws that it was established for the major purpose of developing a chemical standard by which all Aloe vera beverage and cosmetic products could be judged. While NASC continues to exist, at least in name, its 1983 proposed standard was not accepted by the FDA. And, even though the membership voted to accept the standard, very few of its members currently use it. They do not mention the standard in their promotional literature or labeling nor do they make mention of any chemical testing to insure the quality of Aloe vera products or guarantee the concentration of Aloe vera included in any product.

The consumer is, therefore, left on his own as to the facts about Aloe vera, including its uses and its benefits. This anarchy can only be changed if the public demands either that industry wide quality standards be set or that the government set such a standard by vigorous scientific testing in which Aloe vera products are chemically analyzed to insure their quality. Or, the industry might choose to establish a set of rules or standards. This could produce, for example, something like the "Good Housekeeping Seal of Approval."

Even though there is no FDA- approved standard for Aloe vera, it is common knowledge among growers and processors of the plant that Aloe vera juice must be stabilized (preserved in its natural state) to be safe. The FDA further requires that the product be pure, that it must be uncontaminated and unadulterated. Yet, despite the fact that Aloe vera is a vegetable juice, some producers of Aloe vera claim that they have found a way to preserve Aloe without preservatives. The question we must ask here, therefore, is "does that make any sense?" Common sense tells us that it does not.

Aloe vera is no different from any other vegetable juice: if it is sold at room temperature, in plastic containers, or even in glass, then it must have preservatives added or it will rot, just like any other vegetable juice. And, like any other vegetable juice, it can be sold refrigerated, frozen, or even in vacuum sealed cans or containers without the use of preservatives. But that is not how it is being sold at the present time. A complete examination of today's Aloe marketing procedures reveals that almost all Aloe vera juice sold is shipped, stored, and sold at room temperature, mostly in plastic jugs, but also in glass containers. Some of these products bear labels indicating that preservatives and anti-oxidants were used. The labels list the use of preservatives such as sodium benzoate, potassium sorbate, or others, and the use of anti-oxidants such as citric acid, ascorbic acid and others, while some use Vitamin E for this purpose.

Even though there are no chemical standards for Aloe, the FDA requires that Aloe vera juice sold in the United States be free of contaminants. While the FDA does not check Aloe vera products to make sure that they are, in fact, Aloe, they do inspect the facilities of manufacturers of such products and the finished product itself to insure that it is free of contaminants and therefore safe to drink or rub on your skin or use in your mouth or to rub on your head or whatever. In other words these products won't kill you or even make you sick, the prevention of which is the major responsibility of FDA concerning food products and cosmetics.

Do not be misled into believing that Aloe juice sold in plastic containers or even in glass can be sold or handled at room temperature without the use of food preservatives. However, despite this fact, there are many products on the American market which claim to contain no preservatives. Not surprisingly such products generally also look and taste like water. Given the above' facts, any discerning shopper ought to question a product that does not show on its label the use of preservatives which are absolutely necessary if the product is to remain stable and fit for human consumption. Further insight is gained by realizing that water does not need to be preserved. I don't know about you, but I believe that if it looks like water, smells like water, and tastes like water, it is probably water.

DEFINITIONS FOR VARIOUS FORMS OF Aloe vera AS PRESENTED BY THE NATIONAL ALOE SCIENCE COUNCIL IN 1983

RAW Aloe vera GEL -- Naturally occurring, unprocessed, undiluted parenchymal tissue obtained from the decorticated leaves of Aloe Barbadensis Miller (Aloe Vera Linne'), and to which no other material has been added.

100% Aloe vera -- Processed, preserved liquid derived from parenchymal tissue obtained from the decorticated leaves of Aloe Barbadensis Miller (Aloe Vera Linne') containing not more than 50 ppm Aloin and defined by a value of 1000 using the reporting procedure adopted by the NASC.

WHOLE Aloe vera GEL -- Aloe Vera Gel which contains a minimum of 50% of the natural pulp found in Raw Aloe

Vera Gel.

Aloe vera LATEX -- The bitter yellow liquid (sap) contained in the pericyclic tubules of the rind of Aloe Barbadensis Miller, the principle constituent of which is Aloin.

WHOLE LEAF Aloe vera -- Whole leaf of the Aloe Barbadensis Miller including the rind and internal portions of the plant.

ALOE USP -- The dried latex of the leaves of Aloe Barbadensis Miller (Aloe Vera Linne'), known in commerce as Curacao Aloe or Aloe Ferox Miller and hybrids of this species with Aloe Africana Miller and Aloe Spicata Baker known in commerce as Cape Aloe (Fam. Liliaceae).

Aloe vera OIL -- The lipid portion obtained from the leaves of Aloe Barbadensis Miller by various solvent extraction processes.

STABILIZED Aloe vera GEL -- Synonymous with the term Aloe Vera Gel.

Aloe vera PULP -- The parenchymal tissue and fiber derived from Raw Aloe Vera.

Aloe vera CONCENTRATE -- Aloe Vera Gel from which natural water has been mechanically removed and which would have a value of 1500 minimum using the reporting procedure adopted by the NASC.

RECONSTITUTED Aloe vera **GEL** -- Aloe Vera Concentrate to which an appropriate amount of water has been added to achieve a concentration that is equivalent to 100% Aloe Vera as defined above.

Aloe vera **GEL/SPRAY DRIED** -- Aqueous derivative of the leaf of Aloe Barbadensis Miller which has been spray dried on a suitable matrix.

RECONSTITUTED Aloe vera **GEL, SPRAY DRIED** -- Aloe Vera Gel Spray Dried to which an appropriate amount of water has been added to achieve a concentration that is equivalent to 100% Aloe Vera as defined above.

Aloe vera **GEL, FREEZE DRIED** -- Aloe Vera Gel which has been freeze dried with or without a matrix.

RECONSTITUTED Aloe vera **GEL, FREEZE DRIED** -- Aloe Vera Gel Freeze Dried to which an appropriate amount of water has been added to achieve a concentration that is equivalent to 100% Aloe Vera as defined above.

The following are suggested guidelines for nomenclature for edible Aloe Vera:

100% Aloe vera -- Meets the definition of 100% Aloe Vera above. ALOE VERA JUICE -- Product which contains a minimum of 50% Aloe Vera as defined by the procedure adopted by the NASC.

Aloe vera DRINK -- Product which contains a minimum of 10% Aloe Vera as defined by the procedure adopted by the NASC.

Aloe vera EXTRACT -- Product which contains a minimum of 5% Aloe Vera as defined by the procedure adopted by NASC.

Aloe vera FLAVORED -- A Product that contains less than 5% Aloe Vera as defined by the procedure adopted by the NASC.

CHAPTER EIGHT

MISUNDERSTANDING AND CONFUSION

Most writers on the subject of Aloe vera have mindlessly repeated many of the myths already noted in this book. Others, equally as misinformed, claim that there is a native American species of Aloe (making the same mistake as Columbus) or refer to Aloe as a cactus. Still others state that there is only one species of Aloe which has medical value when, as a matter of fact, there are at least three. These three varieties have a large number of common names which has added to the confusion.

Conversely, writers have discussed the fact that there are at least 200 known species or varieties of Aloes; others place the number at 600! Some of these Aloes are only a few inches tall and have leaves as hard as rocks; others are tree size plants over thirty feet tall. However, whatever their number, most of these Aloes have no reported medical value. Sadly, most publications about Aloe vera have done nothing more than confuse the public by making the subject of Aloe much more complicated than it really is. We believe that, in some cases, this has been done deliberately--with misunderstanding and confusion as the ultimate goal. While that may seem like a harsh statement, it is not, for the purpose of such mis-statements has, too often, been to promote and not to inform.

If one uses the pharmaceutical definition of Aloe, then

there are at least three species or varieties of Aloe that deserve the name Aloe vera. They are Aloe vera Linne, Aloe perryi Baker, and Aloe africana Miller.

Aloe vera Linne originated in Northeastern Africa, and is also known by the name, Aloe barbadensis Miller from the Caribbean island of Barbados; hence the sap of this plant is commonly called Barbados Aloes. (In the United States, the use of the "s" on Aloes may be directly responsible for the confusion of references to Aloe(s) in the Bible.) But whatever name is used to identify this species, Aloe vera Linne can be identified by its yellow flower. Many have confused this variety with Aloe chinensis and probably other names world wide. However, Aloe chinensis has an orange flower, while Aloe vera Linne has a yellow flower. And even though Aloe chinensis is reported to have the same medical value, it is probablynot the same variety.

The second major variety is Aloe perryi Baker. In this case the sap is commonly referred to as Socotrine or Curacaon Aloes from the islands of Socotra and Curacao respectively. It is also known as Zanzibar or Cape Aloes. Apparently this is the same as Mocha Aloes which produce a black, pitch-like product and is also known as Jafferabad Aloes. Other names given this variety include Uganda Aloes, Natal Aloes, and Musambra Aloes. In the past many have identified the Aloes referenced by Dioscorides as Socotrine Aloes, but Dioscorides stated that the plants which he used came from India, and this would probably identify the plant used as Aloe vera Linne . Further confusion has been caused by Dioscorides' description of the plant used as having a white flower, although there is no Aloe species which has a truly white flower.

So, one might speculate that Dioscorides either mistakenly stated that his Aloe had a white flower or that the white flowering Aloe has been cross bred out of existence. It is also true that an individual's description of color is highly subjective. There are some species which produce light or pale yellow flowers or even cream colored flowers. Whatever the case, there is no doubt that Dioscorides used Aloe vera. Regardless of the confusion about the flower color of the plant used by Dioscorides, obviously it produced the sap and is therefore a medical Aloe (Aloe vera).

The third species of medical Aloe is Aloe ferox Miller which has a red or reddish-pink flower. Some have also identified this plant as being Aloe Africana Miller. Both of these originated in South Africa, and both are commonly referred to as Cape Aloes. Another variety, Aloe Africana, is often confused with Aloe africana Miller. Aloe Africana has a yellow flower and is therefore not the same species. Even though both may have medical value, Aloe Africana is not officially recognized as being a source of the sap. Some have also further confused the issue by referring to Aloe Africana by many other scientific names including A. spicata, A. platylepia and other names world wide. Actually, the only thing one really needs to understand is that all medical Aloes (Aloe vera) produce a typical bitter yellowish or reddish sap which is their common characteristic.

To add to the confusing history of the Aloe vera plant, some have stated that the Greek word "vera" (which means true or genuine) was used in ancient writings to indicate the use of one specific plant as being better than any other. While it is true that Dioscorides referred to India as being the source of the best Aloes, this was not a declaration that one species of Aloe was better than another for medical purposes, but it simply means that the best quality Aloe (dried sap) came from India. Furthermore, I believe Dioscorides' reference to India was not to the country itself, but rather to a location outside Roman territory, perhaps Cape Verda (modern Somolia) or the island of Soccotra. This theory becomes more plausible when one considers that by the first century A.D., the island of Soccotra had become an important commercial source of the sap. Incidentally, Dioscorides did not use the words "Aloe vera"--that name was not used in ancient times--but was first applied to the plant by Carl Von Linne, a Seventeenth Century Swedish naturalist, who gave the plant its scientific name-- Aloe vera Linne. Linne apparently believed (and so indicated) that he had found a true and genuine Aloe.

Even the origin of the name Aloe has come in for discussion. The word has been traced by some to the Arabic word "alwa" which may be the milk-like, fake Aloe referred to by Pliny the Elder for the word meaning mother's milk. According to Al-Kindi, the Arabic word for Aloe is Sabhra or Sebara. As a point of interest, there is a valley in Lebanon called the Sabhra Valley--a name which is translated as the Valley of the Aloes. It is impossible to prove whether this refers to the growing of Aloe vera in that valley or to the perfume of the Hebrews which came from Aloes trees grown in Lebanon. The final possibility for the derivation of the name is a reference to the Arabic word "Alloeh" which has the meaning "bitter and shiny substance." Of all of the possible sources of the name, this is probably the most plausible. For the ancients used the sap of the plant alone or ground up the whole leaf which, in either case, produced a bitter and shiny substance.

Modern promoters have even made the absurd claim that mixing Aloe with other substances--including water--destroys its function. Since processed Aloe vera is 99 per cent water, one might question how adding water could effect it other than to lower its concentration. The answer is simple; it does not.

A careful look at the historic and scientific documents should convince a discerning student that in ancient times Aloe was routinely mixed with other substances to prepare medicine. On this point researchers and writers have often misstated the content of the Papyrus Ebers. While the Papyrus Ebers gives only general directions for preparation of the leaf (such as grind up and pulverize), it plainly states that Aloe was mixed with other substances such as frankincense, myrrh, honey, juniper berry, mint, unknown green leaves, deerhorn, and others.

Aloe promoters have even misquoted the Materia Medicia of Dioscorides. Indeed, Dioscorides explicitly recommended that Aloe vera be blended with other agents, including water, for use in treating stomach disorders.

During the early 1800's, researchers in the United States began to use tinctures of alcohol to extract the active principles of Aloe, mainly aloin, to be used as laxative or in laxative preparations. By the 1930's and 1940's physicians and scientists were mixing the extracts of the plant with other agents to make the product more appealing to the patient, and apparently all found that these mixing agents had no effect on how Aloe vera worked. For instance, C. E. Wright used the internal contents of the fresh leaf by scraping it out and mixing it with equal amounts of aquaphor to treat x-ray burns. Crewe and Waldon used the insipid juice (sap minus the gel) with lanolin and petrolatum. They later turned to the method of Wright and combined the juice with aquaphor. The practice of mixing Aloe continues today, for instance, in the blending of Aloe with modern sterol cream bases. So it is obvious that the modern myth that adding other substances to Aloe vera hinders its healing abilities has no foundation; the results achieved with such products show that this is a fallacy. As a matter of fact, science and history indicates that the plant (especially the sap) is most useful when mixed with other agents. It also teaches us that the plant provides its own mixing agent--the gel--a point made repeatedly by Collins and Collins, Fine, Rowe, and others over the past 50 years.

Despite the use of the sap as a healing agent in ancient formulary, almost all promoters imply that the sap not only causes allergic reactions but is actually harmful or dangerous, and therefore should not be used in Aloe vera products. In order to sell their products, they have created the myth that the gel alone is the agent of choice, supporting this idea by spreading the untruth that modern studies show the sap is toxic to human tissue or that it causes allergic reactions. Such statements notwithstanding, all published toxicity studies clearly show that Aloe has little or no toxic effects and does not cause allergies. Or perhaps the promoters are simply confused by their superficial understanding of the chemistry of Aloe. To cite only one example of possible misunderstanding is the fact that the sap is scientifically known as an anthraquinone glucoside. According to Merck's Index, an anthraquinone is a <u>synthetic substance</u> used in the manufacture of dyes, which has a systemic toxicity and may cause skin irritation or rashes. Therefore, a poorly informed individual might wrongly conclude from this definition of snythetic anthraquinones, that the sap (which, coincidentally, was and is still used as a dye) is toxic or causes skin rashes or allergic reactions. Perhaps another source of the idea that the plant is toxic or poisonous, is the great Russian encyclopedia, which states that one species of Aloe which grows in Russia is apparently poisonous; however, this species has nothing to do with Aloe vera.

One could go on and on citing examples of mistaken ideas about Aloe vera which have been endlessly repeated by the misinformed. Often specific myths can be traced to their sources of origin. Subsequent writers simply copy the original mistake without any attempt to check the validity of what they repeat, and the confusion is further compounded.

Synergistic Action

During this century, various explanations for the healing effects of Aloe vera have been proposed. Some early researchers theorized that the presence of vitamins--specifically Vitamins A, D and E--were the source of the plant's medical properties. In 1941, this theory was disproved in the paper, "A Phytochemical Study of Aloe vera Leaf," by Tom D. Rowe, who with colleague Lloyd M. Parks, concluded, "The absence of tannin, pectin, vitamin A, vitamin D and the small amount of nitrogenous substances found in the leaf or any concentrated fraction of it, proved that the healing property of Aloe vera leaf is not due to any of these principles or to urea."

Others have proposed that it is the plant's enzymes which are the active agents. This theory is easily dispelled, for when the juice is boiled (long enough to destroy enzymes and vitamins), it still heals. And some have proposed that Aloe's healing properties are due to the amino acids, carbohydrates, simple sugars, water, and minerals of the plant. While it is true that these agents are necessary for good health and the proper healing of damaged tissue, they cannot be either directly or totally responsible. If they were, every fruit and vegetable would demonstrate the same kind of healing effects, since all fruits and vegetables have a chemistry which is very similar to Aloe vera gel. In fact some fruits and vegetables actually contain somewhat higher concentrations of these elements than does Aloe vera gel.

Yet, because we know that the common agents produced or stored by all plants are important in the healing process, it is worth our time to examine their benefits. It is also important to understand the nutritional value of Aloe vera.

Nutritional Value of Aloe vera

Chemical analysis shows that Aloe vera contains vitamins, minerals, triglycerides, carbohydrates, amino acids, enzymes, and, of course, water. The vitamins found in Aloe include B-Complex, B-1, B-2, B-3, Coline, Folic Acid, C, and Carotene (a precursor to Vitamin A)--all of which are vital to general good health in body systems and some of which are vital to the formation of certain enzymes.

Minerals: Aloe has been shown to contain as many as 13 of the 17 minerals needed for good nutrition. Minerals found in Aloe include Calcium, Magnesium, Potassium, Chloride, Iron, Zinc, Manganese, Copper, Chromium, Sulfur, Aluminum and Sodium. All these minerals are vital in the growth process and essential to the function of all body systems.

Triglycerides: Triglycerides include fats, oil and waxes. They carry the fat soluble vitamins, supply the fatty acids essential for growth and general health of all body tissue--especially the skin--and help supply energy.

Carbohydrates: Carbohydrates assist in digestion and assimilation of nutrients in food and supply energy for muscular exertion. They also control protein breakdown, the distribution of sodium, potassium, chloride, water balance, and are essential to healthy skin.

Amino Acids: Aloe vera juice contains twenty of the twenty-two Amino Acids known to be needed for good nutrition; eight or nine of these are essential and must be supplied from an outside source because the body cannot manufacture its own. The other thirteen or fourteen can be built within the body by the essential* eight or nine. Aloe has been shown to contain all of the essential eight or nine. The complete list of Amino acids known to exist in Aloe include *Lysine, *Histidine, *Arginine, Aspartic Acid, Asparagine, *Threonine, Serine, Glutamine, Hydroproline, Proline, Glycine, Alanine, Cystine, *Valine, *Methionine, *Isoledcine, *Leucine, Tyrosine, Glutamis Acid, and *Phenylalanine.

Enzymes: Without enzymes, the chemical reaction of

vitamins, minerals, and hormones cannot take place. Enzymes present in Aloe include Alkaline Phosphatase, Sgotransaminase, Sgptransaminase, Lactic Dehydrogenase, Amylase, Lipase, Oxidase, Peroxidase, Catalase, Bradykininase, Gamma Transaminase, Carboxypeptidase and Cellulase.

Water: Water is the major component of Aloe vera gel (the clear inner part of the leaf.) When the fiber or pulp is removed from the gel, what remains is approximately 99 per cent water. Water is the universal solvent and is responsible for the transfer of nutrients throughout the body.

Some promoters have claimed that Aloe vera gel contains water that is different from the water found in other plants. It is true that the water in plants is cleaner and purer than the water in most cities or municipalities. However, it is a little far-fetched to claim that Aloe vera possesses some sort of magic water--although at least one seller of Aloe whose product looks, smells, and tastes like water, has done just that.

Many researchers have proposed a possible synergistic relationship between all of the substances contained within the Aloe vera plant. Synergistic means the ability of all the chemical and physical components of the plant, working together, to effect a greater benefit than the total sum of each working individually. If correct, this theory might explain the fact that Aloe presents no toxic or allergic effects, even though it contains agents which, if isolated and used alone, can cause toxic and allergic effects. It is obvious that further chemical examination of Aloe vera is required to determine what causes it to work.

In our search for proof of why Aloe works, there are many

sources of information. The first of those references is Rowe's 1941 study mentioned earlier. Although Rowe eliminates the agents already mentioned as being possible sources of the plant's healing effects, he apparently discounted some possible agents which are involved. For example, sulfur and phenols are both mild antiseptics or anti-microbial agents. Rowe identifies the presence of these agents in the rind.

In the 1950's a Russian study discovered the presence of cinnamonic acid and salicylic acid in Aloe vera. These two substances are known anti-microbial agents which are listed as such in major chemical dictionaries. Merck's Index says that cinnamonic acid is an anthelminitic. According to Mosby's Medical Encyclopedia, an anthelminitic is an agent which destroys or prevents infection caused by parasitic worms such as filariae, flukes, hookworms, pinworms, roundworms, schistosomes, tapeworms, trichinae, and whipworms. Perhaps the cinnamonic and salicylic acids and other bacteria present in Aloe vera explains why the Chinese found the plant so effective in treating "worm fevers."

A second report from Russia reports the presence of Traumatic Acid in an extract of Aloe vera used in the treatment of ulcers with excellent results. Traumatic Acid is a wound hormone of plants and is found in the outer rind or skin of many plants. Unfortunately, in the early 1960's, this report was utilized by ulcer researchers in the United States, who incorrectly believed that the source of the Traumatic Acid was the gel of the plant, when, in fact, the agent is in the sap or the rind. The presence of Traumatic Acid in the leaf encourages speculation on its role in healing damaged human skin and tissue (for instance, ulcers).

In 1978, a paper titled "A Chemical Investigation of Aloe Barbadensis Miller" by G. R. Waller, S. Mangiafico and C. R. Ritchey of the Department of Biochemistry, Oklahoma State University, Stillwater, Oklahoma, stated that Aloe barbadensis Miller contains free amino acids, free monosaccharides and total saccharides released upon hydrolysis, sterols, and triterpenoids.

The researchers found that seventeen amino acids, p-glucose, and p-mannose were present in the water-soluble fraction. Cholesterol, campesterol, B-sitosterol, and lupeol were found in substantial amounts in the lipid fraction. An unknown alkaloid(s) was detected using Dragendorff's reagent.

This study identifies a number of compounds which Rowe also found, but the researchers also identify some which Rowe failed to find or did not have the technology to find. Those agents are campesterol, cholesterol, B-sitosterol, and Lupeol. The study states that the leaves examined were dried and that the new compounds were found in the sterol fraction of the leaf. The presence of these agents in Aloe are very important. Campesterol, cholesterol, and B-sitosterol are plant sterols which possess chemical structures which are anti-inflammatory. Lupeol, a hydrochloride, is also an antiseptic and analgesic agent.

In 1982, a University of Chicago Burn Center Report, which will be examined in more detail later in this text, reconfirmed the presence of Salicyclic Acid but adds that this aspirin-like compound is a breakdown product from Aloin (barbaloin) found in the sap. Other researchers have identified the presence of small amounts of Urea Nitrogen, another anti-microbial agent, in the sap.

From the evidence obtained from research, one can postulate that Aloe vera works without toxic or allergic effects because its nutrient and water content act as buffers. The nutrients also are essential to tissue regrowth and function. The plant controls (or eliminates) infections because of natural antiseptic agents -- Sulfur, Phenols, Lupeol, Salicylic Acid, Cinnamonic Acid, and Urea Nitrogen. It controls inflammation due to its anti-inflammatory fatty acids, Cholesterol, Campesterol, and B-sitosterol, and it limits or stops pain because of its content of Lupeol, Salicylic Acid and Magnesium. Acting together, these agents and the leaves' others agents constitute that synergistic relationship. Thus we see a rational explanation for the numerous reports that Aloe vera eliminates many internal and external infections, limits or eliminates inflammation, and is a highly effective pain killer. Chemistry explains Aloe's ability to work as an effective treatment for burns, cuts, scrapes, and abrasions as well as for the treatment of many inflammatory conditions such as rheumatic fever, arthritis of all kinds, disorders of the skin, mouth, esophagus, stomach, small intestine, colon, and other internal organs such as the kidney, spleen, pancreas, and liver.

It is important to remember that the anti-inflammatory and anti-bacterial agents are found in the sap and the rind of the plant, not in the gel. At the same time one must not forget that the basic nutrients and other agents are widely dispersed throughout the plant--meaning the sap, the gel, and the rind --and about 98 per cent of the water is confined to the gel. This knowledge should help put pseudo-scientific fallacies to rest, especially the widely held myth that the gel of the plant is totally responsible for the healing ability of Aloe vera. At the same time, we need to avoid an overreaction which dismisses the gel as worthless. The gel is important as a buffering agent. Therefore, the theory of a synergistic relationship is the one which is supportable with both history and science.

At this point in our search for the truth, we have a chemical explanation of Aloe vera's ability to heal through its capabilities to control or kill a number of disease-causing microbes, to alleviate (or eliminate) pain, and to counteract inflammation.

We know that it has been repeatedly stated that the plant has all of these abilities, and more. As yet, we have not even mentioned Aloe vera's reported ability to eliminate excessive water from tissue, to aid digestion, to balance body acidity, to eliminate or greatly reduce scarring, to regenerate hair follicles, to return injured or damaged skin to its normal, healthy color, or many other benefits that will be explored as we move from the theoretical back to the practical.

Analytical Profile of Aloe Vera leaves as presented by the National Aloe Science Council in 1983

To develop the standardizing information, as shown at the end of this chapter, samples of fresh Aloe vera leaf and processed Aloe vera juice or gel were gathered from various growers, processors, and manufacturers from the Rio Grande Valley of Texas over a ten-month period (from September, 1981 to July, 1982).

The fresh leaf was processed and chemical analysis was

performed on it and all of the samples (approximately 250). As demonstrated by the Analytical Profile of Aloe vera Leaves, thirty components and three other factors were considered as being sufficient to define Aloe vera juice. Of these, the percentage of solids (material other than water and juice) calcium and magnesium plus an HPLC Ratio were considered stable enough factors to define the juice. Using these four, a mathematical formula was proposed by the technical committee of National Aloe Science Council (NASC) and was accepted by the membership.

This formula stated that 100 per cent Aloe vera juice would have a mathematical value of 1,000. The formula was then presented to the FDA in early 1983. FDA swiftly rejected the mathematical formula, stating that one could not define Aloe vera juice this way. FDA added that they would consider a product to be 100 per cent Aloe vera juice if it had no more than 10 per cent added water and it was preserved (stabilized) with approved food additives.

After extensive examination of the standard (which consists of thirty-three factors), this writer concluded that the standard itself could be used to determine that a product was not Aloe vera but could not emphatically be used to prove that a product was, in fact, Aloe vera. In other words, if a product that claims to be Aloe vera and does not contain the agents listed at, or near, the levels shown under minimums, it is almost certain that it is not 100% Aloe vera. If the levels are below the minimums (poorest quality individual sample tested), then water has probably been added, but it is also possible that the leaf was grown under poor conditions. If a product does not contain any agents shown, then it is not Aloe vera, period.

The analytical profile of Aloe vera leaf also shows a maximum (best sample tested) and an average column (average of all samples tested). If one applies the (NASC) mathematical formula to the numbers in the minimum column, a reading of 857.35 or 85.735 per cent Aloe vera is obtained. Doing the same to the maximum column, one achieves a reading of 1861.8 or 186.18 per cent Aloe vera. If applied to the average column, a reading of 1169.78 or 116.978 per cent Aloe vera is shown. Unfortunately, here too, we find a problem which is that the formula is valid if one knows for certain that the product being tested, is, in fact, Aloe vera. It should be obvious, however, that blinding using the NASC information alone, could lead one to mistakenly identify any vegetable or fruit juice as Aloe vera gel. Since almost all the 33 factors are common to all vegetable and fruit juices. But there is one factor that is not common, which is the HPLC Ration. According to the NASC, this ration examines the presence of barbatol in Aloe vera. The word barbatol is used as a synonym for Barbaloin which is the sap. In other words, once again, the factor that separates Aloe from other vegetable juice, is the presence of the sap.

But here too we find confusion because, according to NASC, the standard was developed to verify that a product was Aloe vera gel or contained Aloe vera gel that did not contain the sap. So, it seems the NASC want to have their cake and eat it too, stating that the standard formula is a test for the gel alone but make its major factor the presence of the sap.

Analytical Profile of Aloe vera Leaves

TEST	UNITS	MINIMUM	MAXIMUM	AVERAGE
Solids	%	0.75	1.50	0.92
Water	%	98.5	99.25	99.1
Glucose	mg/dl	28.0	103.0	77.8
Purine	mg/dl	0.1	5.6	0.8
Urea-Nitrogen	mg/dl	1.0	1.0	1.0
Creatinine	mg/dl	0.1	1.5	0.4
Sodium	meq/l	4.0	13.0	8.7
Potassium	meq/l	10.0	22.5	13.4
Chloride	meq/l	1.0	11.0	3.0
CO2	meq/l	1.0	7.0	1.7
Calcium	mg/dl	19.4	48.5	30.0
Cal. Calcium	mg/dl	23.3	52.3	33.8
Magnesium	mg/dl	3.2	4.7	3.9
Zinc	mg/dl	14.0	77.0	31.0
Phosphorus	mg/dl	0.6	1.3	1.0
Total Protein	gm/dl	0.1	0.4	0.2
Albumin	gm/dl	0.1	0.5	0.14
Globulin	gm/dl	0.0	2.0	0.06
Alkaline Phosphatase	mg/dl	1.0	50.0	18.0
Sgotransaminase	mg/dl	6.0	49.0	21.0
Sgptransaminase	mg/dl	8.0	85.0	24.0
Lactic Dehydrogenase	mg/dl	0.0	9.0	3.0
Amylase	mg/dl	0.0	2.0	1.0
Lipase	units/dl	0.0	1.6	0.5
Cholestrol	mg/dl	4.0	12.0	8.0
Triglycerides	mg/dl	1.0	12.0	2.4
Iron	meg/dl	3.0	30.0	15.0
B12	pg/ml	141.0	403.0	265.0
Folic Acid	ng/ml	2.7	20.0	13.2
Osmolarity	mOsm/kg	43.0	67.0	60.0
HPLC Ratio		0.51	1.1	0.67

The chart above shows the components found in Aloe vera & the HPLC ratio as reported by the N.A.S.C. in 1983.

CHAPTER NINE

TOXICOLOGY

In "The Overselling of Aloe vera," the FDA leaves a troubling, open-ended question when the article's author indicates concern that Aloe vera juice, if ingested, may be toxic. At the same time, the author notes that a 1974 study showed that Aloe vera juice was not toxic to rats.

As a matter of fact, a perusal of the literature concerned with the possible toxicity of Aloe vera shows that not only is Aloe NOT TOXIC BUT THAT IT ACTUALLY PROMOTES TISSUE REGENERATION.

Oddly enough, in 1959, the FDA itself apparently concluded that Aloe was not toxic. Or at least that is the impression left by Gunnar Gjerstad and T.D. Riner in their article "Current Status of Aloe As A Cure-All." Gjerstad and Riner reviewed data submitted by E. P. Pendergrass concerning the effectiveness of Aloe as a treatment for X-ray and other radiation burns and admitted that the Aloe ointment used by Pendergrass actually regenerated skin tissue.

The rest of this chapter will attempt to answer the question, "Is Aloe vera toxic; that is, does it kill tissue or does it actually regenerate tissue? Although there is a large body of anecdotal evidence that Aloe heals and regenerates living tissue, the question is still being asked by those who need more proof than positive results. In other words, the doubters want specific studies done to show that Aloe does not kill living tissue and that it regenerates living tissue.

One such study was published by Hazleton Laboratories, Inc., a subsidiary of TRW, Inc., Falls Church, VA, in January, 1969. The issue of toxicity was addressed in their paper, "13-Week Repeated Dermal Application--Rabbits--Stabilized Aloe vera Gel-- Final Report."

The researchers at Hazleton concluded that repeated applications of Aloe vera did not result in histopathologic changes in any of the tissues examined. Nor did Aloe cause any "related histopathological alterations in the liver, kidney, or skin of albino rabbits." In other words, Aloe vera is not toxic.

Also from 1969 is Dr. E. R. Zimmerman's article "The Effects of Prednisolone, Indomethacin, and Aloe vera Gel on Tissue Culture Cells" in Federal Dental Services. Zimmerman says that after using Aloe vera in various concentrations, it was determined that Aloe vera was less toxic than Prednisolone or Indomethacin when tested on the Gey strain of HeLa cells and rabbit kidney fibroblasts. It is worth noting that this study concluded that Aloe vera caused the living cells studied to live up to two-thirds longer than would normally be expected! So not only did Aloe not kill the cells, it actually encouraged them to live in a thriving condition longer.

As the use of Aloe vera as a tonic or beverage becomes more popular, the alert consumer is rightfully asking if drinking Aloe could possibly be harmful. Furthermore, since real 100 percent Aloe to drink is not cheap, he is wondering if any real benefit is to gained by regularly drinking the product.

This question was addressed by Jeffrey Bland. Ph.D. in an

article in <u>Prevention Magazine </u>in March-April 1985. Dr. Bland, of the Linus Pauling Institute of Science and Medicine, Palo Alto, CA in his medical paper, "Effect of Orally Consumed Aloe vera Juice on Gastrointestinal Function In Normal Humans," studied ten healthy individuals, five men (average age 42) and five women (average age 32). The study did not require any of the individuals studied to change their diet or lifestyle, other than to consume two ounces of Aloe vera juice three times daily for seven consecutive days, and to eat a meal replacement bar at breakfast.

The semi-controlled study required the test subjects to fast overnight before entering the study for purposes of evaluation of their gastricsecretion which was measured by a pH sensitive capsule that transmitted information to a receiver worn around the waist. A stool sample and morning urine sample were taken after completion of the capsule pH study. The urine and stool were examined to determine if the Aloe had any unusual effects on these two bodily secretions.

The report states, "Evaluation of the data collected on each subject before and after Aloe vera juice supplementation produced information on the average changes in urinary changes in urinary indican, stool specific gravity, gastric pH, and bowel mobility. (See Tables 1 through 4 at the end of this chapter .) As can be seen from Table 1, urinary indican values were seen to decrease, on the average one full unit, after Aloe vera juice intake for one week. This is indicative of lowered bowel bacterial conversion of tryptophan and possibly improved protein digestion and absorption after the Aloe vera juice treatment."

"Increased urinary indican is reflective of reduced protein

digestion and absorption and increased bowel putrefaction of the amino acid tryptophan, (8) and the lower value of urinary indican seen after the Aloe vera juice supplementation trial, suggests improved protein digestion assimilation with reduced bacterial putrefaction."

The study goes on to say that the specific gravity of the stool was reduced an average of 0.37 with faster movement of the stool through the digestive system, both suggesting an increase in the amount of water in the stool. Further noted is the fact that this caused the test subjects' digestion to move toward what is considered more normal, and no diarrhea was reported. Also noted was the fact that Aloe acts as a buffering agent which helps to normalize the pH--that is, acts as an alkalyzing agent.

Furthermore, according to Dr. Bland, the use of Aloe helped to normalize the stool cultures in six subjects, four of the six having high amounts of yeast, which was greatly reduced, indicating that Aloe promotes a more favorable balance of gastrointestinal symbiotic bacteria. Five of the subjects suffered from indigestion, irritable bowel syndrome, colitis, and excess acid stomach, and all five reported relief from these conditions by the oral administration of Aloe vera juice. The report notes that these findings support the previously acknowledged bacteriostatic properties of Aloe vera juice applied topically.

In discussing his findings, Dr. Bland stated, "The tolerance of the subjects to Aloe vera juice supplementation was in general, quite good. One subject complained of gas and another of transient gut pain, which after continued supplementation throughout the week, diminished. The other eight subjects were asymptomatic with no diarrhea, nausea, intestinal bloating, or distress. Four of the subjects noted an improved bowel regularity with greater gastrointestinal comfort after eating. Three of the subjects indicated that they felt some enhancement of energy and a sense of well-being, although this could not be confirmed quantitatively."

Interestingly enough, in all three of these studies, the Aloe vera used was provided by the same grower, processor, and manufacturer, and was yellow in color and had a somewhat disagreeable odor and a bitter taste. The Aloe had been pasteurized and contained preservatives--the very sort of product which in recent years has seen a decline in sales, but more recently has begun to re-emerge as a popular product because the consumer is beginning to learn that if an Aloe vera product looks like water...it does not work.

At the risk of being redundant, we have stated repeatedly that real Aloe vera does not look like water. We have deliberately emphasized this fact because even if the consumer has no other information by which to judge the quality of the Aloe drink product he is buying, then the products appearance is the consumer's first line of defense against being misled or defrauded. So, if an Aloe vera drink is not yellowish or reddish, what you are buying is not Aloe vera, regardless of what the seller claims.

Table 1

Urinary Indican Levels Before and After Aloe Vera Trial

Subject	Sex	Before*	After*
N.M.	F	Trace	Trace
P.S.	F	2	Negative
L.Z.	F	Trace	Trace
S.G.	F	4	1
S.M.	F	3	2
L.B.	M	1	2
P.M.	M	4	1
M.A.	M	1	Trace
J.B.	M	3	2
J.F.	M	3	3

Average change - 1.0 indican units
*Values rated from zero to 4; highest indican = 4

Table 2

Stool Specific Gravity Before and After Aloe Vera Trial

Subject	Sex	Before*	After*
N.M.	F	0.92	0.92
P.S.	F	1.27	1.00
L.Z.	F	1.50	1.25
S.G.	F	1.43	1.07
S.M.	F	2.70	1.30
L.B.	M	2.20	1.70
P.M.	M	1.44	1.08
M.A.	M	1.18	1.00
J.B.	M	1.12	1.10
J.F.	M		

Average change - 0.3 after aloe treatment

Table 3

Gastric pH One Hour After the Administration of the Meal Replacement Bar

Subject	Sex	Before*	After*
N.M.	F	1.4	3.4
P.S.	F	3.2	4.1
L.Z.	F	3.2	4.0
S.G.	F	3.1	5.4
S.M.	F	3.2	5.3
L.B.	M	2.7	4.0
P.M.	M	1.6	4.7
M.A.	M	4.2	4.5
J.B.	M	3.2	4.1
J.F.	M	4.1	4.7

Average change after aloe vera administration + 1.88 pH units

---

Table 4

Time of Capsule Transfer to Duodenum and Stool Culture Effects of Aloe Vera

Subject	Sex	Change in time of capsule to duodenum	Qualitative effect of Aloe on Stool Culture
N.M.	F	-1	No difference
P.S.	F	0	Lowered yeast
L.Z.	F	0	Lowered bacteria
S.G.	F	+1	No dfference
S.M.	F	-2	Lowered bacteria
L.B.	M	0	Lowered yeast
P.M.	M	-2	Lowered yeast
M.A.	M	-1	No difference
J.B.	M	0	No difference
J.F.	M	-1	Lower yeast

Preventive Medicine, March/April 1985

CHAPTER TEN

RESEARCH AND REPORTS 1934-1988

According to "Webster's New Collegiate Dictionary," MEDICINE is "A substance or preparation used in treating disease; something that affects well-being; the science and art dealing with the maintenance of health and the prevention, alleviation, or cure of disease; the branch of medicine concerned with the non-surgical treatment of disease; a substance (as a drug or potion) used to treat something other than disease; an object held by the American Indians to give control over natural or magical forces; magical power or a magical rite."

As we have already seen in our review of the history of Aloe vera as a medicinal plant, it was not until 1934 that the first modern medical study on Aloe's ability to heal was published in the United States by C.E. Collins. Collins and his son then wrote a second paper on the use of Aloe vera in the treatment of radiation injury and reported over 50 patients treated with Aloe vera.

Both papers, reviewed the case of a 31-year- old female patient with severe roentgen dermatitis. Although the reports of Collins and Collins are perfectly clear, several authorities have asserted that Aloe vera probably had nothing to do with the recovery of the woman in question but have asserted that she was frightened into healing herself because of her fear of the alternate method of treatment, skin grafts. So she healed herself, these learned men of science claimed.

Collins and Collins described the condition of the patient in question, "There was a desquamation over an area 4 by 8 cm. on the left side of the forehead, extending 2 cm. above the hair line. The medical history showed that in May, 1932, she had received (in another city) what she had been told was a depilatory x-ray treatment. Fourteen months later, she said, the skin of the forehead and scalp became rough and scaby, and itched continuously (dermatitis exfoliativa). Between July, 1933, and March, 1934, she had successively consulted three physicians, all of whom had agreed as to the diagnosis and who had prescribed (variously) boric acid, phenol in olive oil, ichthyol, a 5 per cent mercurial ointment, and zinc oxide. The condition had become progressively worse until there was (as has been stated) extensive desquamation with oozing of serious fluid.

The patient stated that the itching and burning sensations were so severe and constant that she was compelled to wear cotton gloves at night in order to prevent scratching the damaged area, and inducing bleeding. After a review of this history and an examination of the condition, it was felt that a skin graft was indicated, and the patient was so advised. At the time of examination the patient was furnished with a quantity of Aloe vera (fresh whole leaf) for local application, with the hope that this material might serve as a palliative (i.e. act to allay the itching). Twenty-four hours later she reported, that the sensations of itching and burning had entirely subsided. She was instructed to continue the use of the plant material, and when seen from time to time during the next five weeks the condition was found to be progressively improved.

"At the end of this time (i.e. on April 7, 1934), there was complete regeneration of the skin of the forehead and scalp, new hair growth, complete restoration of sensation, and absence of scar. There was at this time a slight blanching of the affected area. When last seen on July 23, 1934, the healed area appeared to be completely cured, with no indication whatever of a relapse. On exposure to the summer sunlight the forehead skin was seen to be pigmenting normally along with other exposed skin surfaces of the body."

Collins said the results achieved in this case encouraged him to use Aloe vera on a few cases of raydermatitis. He concludes the report by saying, "Since April, 1934, we have treated more than fifty cases of x-ray and radium burns with Aloe vera leaf and ointment, known as "Alvagel," made from the leaf. While all have not been perfect cures, the results as a whole have been most gratifying."

In 1936, Dr. Carroll S. Wright, M.D., Philadelphia, in his medical paper, "Aloe Vera in the Treatment of Roentgen Ulcers and Telangiectasis," published in the Journal of the American Medical Association, Vol. 106, reported on his use of Aloe vera to treat several patients in the manner suggested by Collins. Although Wright had received a personal communication from Creston Collins in 1934," ...in which he warned me that results could not be expected in x-ray squelae of more than two years' duration.' I began the use of the fresh Aloe vera leaf in the treatment of two cases of x-ray telangiectasia resulting from ill advised attempts at x-ray depilation by local advertising concerns, and in one case of radium telangiectasia of ten years' duration. Because of the difficulty of applying the whole leaf directly to the areas in question, I scraped out the intestional contents of the Aloe vera leaf and mixed it with an equal quantity of aquaphor and had the patient massage this into the skin every night.

Wright continues, "The Aloe vera leaf contains a large quantity of light yellowish green material having about the color and consistency of lemon "Jello" [sic]; it is the intestinal material that is used for local applications. The directions given by C. E. and Creston Collins are to spread the leaf lengthwise or cut it into thick cross sections, macerate the intestinal material, and while it is still fresh to apply liberal quantities to the area to be treated, covering it with a neutral, nonporous substance such as waxed paper. A bandage is used to keep it in place."

Wright reported that, "Since October, 1934, seven cases of x-ray telangiectasia and the one case of radium telangiectasia have been treated by this method...No improvement was obtained as regards the degree of telangiectasia but the texture of the skin was improved in all cases.

"My purpose in this case is to present the remarkable improvement obtained in two cases of x-ray ulceration with the hope of stimulating interest in what promises to be a revolutionary method of treatment for early x-ray damage to the skin and ulceration of the skin resulting from x-rays."

In November, 1936, Adolph B. Loveman, M.D., of Louisville, KY, in his medical paper on "Leaf of Aloe Vera in Treatment of Roentgen Ray Ulcers," reported on two additional cases in which treatment with Aloe vera was noted. Dr. Loveman stated that he used Aloe in much the same way that

Collins and Collins had noted earlier.

The first patient Loveman reported on was a man aged 40, suffering from severe roentgen raydermatitis involving the backs of both hands. Like Collins and Collins, Loveman stated that many other methods of treatment had been tried unsuccessfully. On the advise of Dr. Oliver Ormsby, treatment with fresh Aloe vera was started on March 11, 1936. It took almost two and one half weeks to relieve the pain and approximately five weeks to see any definite signs of healing. However, Loveman concludes by saying, that by November, 1936, the entire ulceration had healed, although there were still a few keratoses and sclerotic areas. The texture of the skin, however, had been markedly improved.

The second patient was a male, 46 years of age, who suffered a severe dermatitis involving both hands. Treatment with the fresh whole leaf of Aloe vera was started March 3, 1936. In this case the patient was free from pain within 36 hours, healing was obvious in a few days, and was complete by May 27, 1936.

In 1938, Archie Fine, M.D., and Samuel Brown, M.D., Cincinnati, OH, in their medical paper, "Cultivation and Clinical Application of Aloe Vera Leaf," Tumor Clinic and the Department of Roentgenology, respectively, Jewish Hospital, reported on the use of fresh whole Aloe vera leaf in the treatment of radiology burns. They said, "We have noted in those cases which are receiving prolonged courses of therapy whereby the skin is becoming irritated and painful, though intact, that application of the leaf is extremely soothing, and allays the discomfort considerably. This was noted especially in breast (cancer) cases, in which the axilla received a large amount of radiation and became quite painful.

"Interesting enough, the gardener in charge of the greenhouse (from which the researchers obtained their Aloe vera) informed us that he had cultivated Aloes more than fifty years ago in Europe, and was well-acquainted with the plant's value in the treatment of pruritic skin lesions."

In 1939, Dr. Frederick B. Mandeville, M.D., Professor of Radiology, Medical College of Virginia, Richmond, VA in his medical paper, "Aloe vera in the Treatment of Radition Ulcers of Mucous Membranes," reported on his successful use of Aloe vera in the treatment of five cases and stated, "All five (of the patients) have experienced definite relief from pain and discomfort..."

According to Dr. Mandeville, "One case of severe roentgen dermatitis of the face, treated two years ago with the fresh leaf, can be recorded as an excellent result. Three other cases of roentgen ulcers of the skin, in patients treated for carcinomas of the prostate, breast, and vagina, died incidently to their disease, before a reasonably accurate or satisfactory evaluation of Aloe vera therapy could be made. Relief from pain was definite, sloughing appeared to clear more readily, and skin grafting was successful in the breast cast."

In 1940, Tom D. Rowe, in his medical paper, "A Preliminary Report the Effect of Fresh Aloe vera Jell in the Treatment of Third-Degree Roentgen Reactions on White Rats," reported on a controlled study of the use of fresh Aloe vera leaf on five groups of rats. He said, "One year after the last group had been treated, 13 of the rats were living. One of these was from the check control group. All the others had been treated with the jell (Aloe vera). Of these, both areas showed complete macroscopic healing on nine rats. A small...scab was present on the treated area of one rat, the treated area being completely healed."

Rowe concluded, "To date, no definite conclusions have been drawn from the work because: (1) too few animals have received treatment; (2) the 14-day period of treatment is too short a time on which to base final conclusions.

From the results obtained, fresh Aloe vera jell shows some promise of being of value in the treatment of X- ray reactions. Plans have been made to continue this problem along the lines already pursued. A larger number of animals is to be treated for a longer period of time."

In October, 1941, Rowe, B. K. Lovell, and Lloyd M. Parks published a second medical paper titled, "Further Observations on the Use of Aloe vera Leaf in the Treatment of Third Degree X-Ray Reactions," and published in the Journal of the American Pharmaceutical Association. Rowe, Lovell and Parks came to the conclusion, "Sufficient data have been obtained to show that treatment with the pulp of the leaf definitely increases the rate of healing of such experimentally produced reactions. Furthermore, contrary to previous views, our results indicate that the pulp does not have to be fresh in order to be effective as a healing agent."

In August, 1945, in the American Review of Soviet Medicine, V. P. Filatov, in his medical paper on "Tissue Therapy in Cutaneous Leishmaniasis," reported on successful use of Aloe vera in seven cases of Cutaneous Leishmaniasis.

In 1947, in a paper published in the American Journal of Botany, T. C. Barnes, Hahneunan Medical College and

Hospital of Philadelphia, PA. reported on the successful use of fresh Aloe vera leaf mixed with petrolatum in the treatment of self-inflicted wounds to the tips of the fingers created with sterile sandpaper. He said Aloe vera will cause healing at a rate of at lest one-third faster than would normally be expected.

In 1953, C. C. Lushbaugh, M.D., and D. B. Hale, B.S., in their medical paper published in <u>Cancer,</u> Vol. 6 (No. 4), and titled "Experimental Acute Radiodermatitis Following Beta Irradiation, A V. Histopathological Study of the Mode of action of Therapy with Aloe vera," said, "These experiments show objectively that Aloe vera has a remarkably curative effect upon radiodermatitis in the rabbit. It was found to increase greatly the development of the lesion by apparently doing away with the so-called latent period."

Lushbaugh and Hale claimed, "Treatment was found to hasten both the degenerative and reparative phases of the lesion so that complete healing of an ulcer caused by 28,000 rep of beta radiation was accomplished within two months of treatment, while the untreated ulcerations were still not completely healed more than four months after radiation. The researchers concluded that Aloe vera contains substances that are stimulating both to the delayed development and delayed healing of ulcerative radiodermatitis and that because of the growing modern importance of this injury, further investigation of the action of Aloe vera should be pursued."

In 1956-57, a very interesting study was done by N. Nordvinov and B. Rostotsky of the Radiological Department of the State Research Roentgeno-Radiological Institute of the RSFSR Ministry of Health and the Chemical Department of the All-Union Research Institute of Medicinal and Aromatic Plants. In their medical paper, "Comparison of the Effectiveness of the Juice of Aloe Arborescens with the Juice of Aloe Striatula for the Phophylayis of Radiation Injuries," they state that the Aloe emulsion, "is one of the most effective preparations when tested on radiation therapy of 200 patients with various...malignant tumors."

They go on to say that the emulsion is recommended "for preventing the development of local reactions in radiation therapy, in the treatment of dry and moist epidermititis and treating radiation burns of the 2nd and 3rd degrees, in gynecology--in the treatment of kraurosis vulvae (a skin disease of aged women characterized by dryness, itching, and atrophy of the vulva.) The condition often leads to cancer. (Source: Mosby Medical Encyclopedia, 1985), in cases of eczema, psoriasis, neurodermititis, lichen rubber planus and other skin diseases.) Aloe emulsion was successfully administered also in a number of other disorders, particularly for heat burns, frostbite, for treating cuts, blisters, etc."

They conclude by stating that the emulsion reduced the sensitivity of the skin to ionizing irradiation, and noted a reduction in time for healing to occur (epithelization) from 30-45 days to 15-16 days, indicating that Aloe vera greatly speeds the healing process.

In 1956-57, S. Levenson and K. Somova, Therapeutic Stomatology, Irkukak Medical Institute, Russia, in on "Periodontosis (Disease of the Bond Holding Teeth) Treated with Aloe Extract," stated that Aloe extract was used for the treatment of periodontitis (disease which destroys the bonding of the teeth to the bones within the gum--Mosby's Medical Encyclopedia, a 1985) and subgingival and supergingival dental calculus (small mineral deposits on the gum next to the teeth or actually on the teeth--Mosby's Medical Encyclopedia, 1985). The study notes that more than 150 patients, both men and women, were treated, by injecting a solution of Aloe mixed with 1 ml of a 0.5% procaine hydrochloride at the site of each affected tooth. The course of treatment included 30 injections with a five day interval following the 15th injection.

"The following was observed: 3-4 injections reduced bleeding from the gums, itching of the gums disappears; 6-8 injections result in the appearance of secretion from the pathological gum pockets, the unpleasant taste and odor in the mouth disappear, as well as the nagging toothache. After 12-15 injections, the patients indicate a sensation of freshness in the oral cavity and a feeling of stability of the teeth."

The study concludes by stating that normal color returned to all gum tissue and edema disappeared. Further, the membrane around the tooth was tightened to help strengthen the support for loose teeth. Besides that, the number of lymphhocytes in the blood drops to normal as a result of treatment with Aloe vera.

In conclusion, they noted, "In 75% of periodontosis patients, the number of lymphocytes increased. The number of lymphocytes returns to normal under the effect of treatment with biogenic stimulation. The reduction in the number of lymphocytes to normal is, to a certain extent, an objective indication of treatment results."

In April, 1963, in the Journal of the American Osteopathic Association, Vol.62, by Julian J. Blitz, D.O., James W.

Smith, D.O., and Jack R. Gerard, D. O., Dania, FL, in their medical paper, "Aloe vera Gel in Peptic Ulcer Therapy: Preliminary Report," said that they used Aloe vera gel as the sole medication (except in isolated instances in which Pro-Banthine was used for overwhelming distress that indicated the need for the immediate restraint of hydrochloric acid secretion) for the treatment of peptic ulcers in eighteen patients. They state that all patients had completely recovered by 1961, except an 18-year-old female who only received a few treatments and never returned to the clinic.

The researchers stated, "Clinically, Aloe vera gel emulsion has dissipated all symptoms in patients considered to have incipient peptic ulcer. Duodenitis, probably representing duodenal ulcer but lacking x-ray demonstration of pathognomonic deformity, treated with Aloe vera gel, resulted in uniformly excellent recovery, except questionably in one patient. In case of peptic ulcer about which there could be little clinical doubt, and in every instance confirmed by roentgenologic identification of a flick, niche, or crater with accompanying hypermotile manifestations, Aloe vera gel emulsion provided complete recovery."

In 1973, a medical paper was published in Dermatology, January- February issue, Vol. 12 No. 1, titled "Use of Aloe in Treating Leg Ulcers and Dermatoses," and was authored by M. El Zawahry, M.D., Professor of Dermatology, Faculty of Medicine, Cairo University; M. Rashad Hegazy, M.D., head, Pharmacology Department, Nile Company for Pharmaceuticals, Cairo; and M. Helal, B.Ph., Ph.Ch., head, Phytochemistry Department, Nile Company for Pharmaceuticals, Cairo.

These physicians began their medical report in a way which is very common to such papers, giving us a brief history of the use of the Aloe vera plant, but in so doing, they repeated at least two of the most common myths about the plant and its history...the idea that there are drawings of the Aloe vera plant found on Egyptian temple walls and that Hippocrates described Aloe vera and its medicinal uses. As already mentioned, neither of these myths are true.

It is important to point out that these fine doctors unfortunately attempted to totally remove the gel (from the sap) by cutting the base of the leaf off and allowing the leaf to drain for a period of 48 hours. However, based on the results achieved in this study, it is obvious that they overlooked the fact that the process of draining the sap from the leaf did not eliminate it from the product used in their tests.

This is borne out when they state, "Aloe vera contains a bitter substance, aloin, present in the pericycle and gelatinous material forming the pulp of the leaves." This points directly to the fact that the product used here contained the sap, the only part of the leaf that is bitter. The gel has almost no taste, little color, almost no odor, that is, unless the sap is present.

The Cairo study reports on three cases of chronic leg ulcerations. The first patient was a fifty-year-old merchant, who "stood during his work, had chronic varicose ulcers on the left leg of 15 years' duration, surrounded by eczema, otherwise he was in good health.

"The patient had a large ulcer on the medial surface of about 1400 millimeters square...and a smaller one on the lateral surface of the left leg. The ulcers were deep, foul-smelling and their bases were dirty and fixed. The margins were irregular."

The report states that healing began within one week, and after six weeks the lateral ulcer was completely healed. After ten weeks the crust on the lateral ulcer fell off and the wound was completely healed. The medial ulcer went through approximately the same healing process, but took approximately eleven weeks to completely heal.

The second patient, a man aged fifty-one, had edema and pseudolephantiasis of the left leg and foot with roughness and corrugation of the skin. He had chronic and foul- smelling leg ulcers of seven years' duration, a huge one on the back of the left leg of about 5000 millimeters square, and two smaller ulcers on the medial surface of the same leg, an upper and a lower one. Unlike the first patient, the second patient complained of throbbing pain during the first two weeks of treatment when the leg was lowered, but this pain had disappeared after two weeks. The small ulcers healed within six weeks; the larger showed vast improvement within nine weeks , and even though the report is inconclusive, it appears that ultimate healing did occur. It was noted that the surface of this ulcer did begin to bleed as circulation was improved.

The third case, a twenty-two year old man, had suffered a burn on the medial lower left leg eight years previous, and an ulcer developed on the burn site five years later. The doctors state that, "Five months before he came to us, it became painful with pain increasing on standing. He had varicose veins in the leg, with pigmentation of skin around the ulcer.

"The ulcer had an area of about four hundred and forty square millimeters. It was dirty with purulent effusion and necrotic material at the bottom of the lower part.

"After five weeks of Aloe treatment there was good progress of healing of the ulcer and the epithelium moved toward the inside. The area progressively decreased during treatment."

In discussing their results, the doctors note that there was no effective treatment for ulcers available at the time of the report, thus making the point that any treatment showing promise was a great advance. They also note that the Aloe had improved the circulation in the ulcerated areas, a statement which is supported by numerous other doctors in their respective medical papers.

They further stated, "We believe that the active principle for promoting healing is mucopolysaccharides which are present in high concentration in Aloe gel. Authors note: Here again, it is obvious the doctors mean a combination of gel and sap.

In a second study, prompted by the results of their initial work, the Egyptian doctors investigated the effects of Aloe in cases of seborrhea, acne and alopecia, suggesting the healing capacity of Aloe vera in chronic leg ulcers encouraged them to use it for alopecia and hair fall.

The researchers believed that if Aloe were used in treatment of these problems, it would be necessary to use it for a long period of time. They went on to state that Aloe decreased the loss of hair and completely stopped it from falling by the end of the first month, a common factor in all three patients examined. Two of the patients had shown re-growth of hair in bald areas within three months. Treatment had a positive effect on the patient's seborrhea when applied topically.

A further study of hair loss was conducted on other patients with a variety of alopecia. One group of three patients showed rapid initiation of hair growth; "One of them, a boy aged 12 years, had hair growing in the alopecia area within one week. Ten patients with different etiological causes of their hair fall are now being treated and the preliminary reports are encouraging."

This trio of doctors went on to treat three women between the ages of twenty and twenty-five for mixed acne vulgaris. The doctors noticed that drying of the face preceded improvement in all cases. At one month, treatment resulted in two of the three being totally free of acne and the third showing marked improvement, with little signs of acne remaining.

"No patient treated with Aloe vera had untoward reaction," they continued, "No case of contact dermatitis was reported. No active irritation happened to any of the treated patients with seborrhea, acne vulgaris or alopecia. Control cases were few, one for each disease, but no control patient was affected by the vehicle alone."

In summary, they said, "Aloe vera proved to have a stimulating effect on the rate of healing of chronic leg ulcers. We believe improvement in three patients treated can be attributed to improvement in the peripheral circulation which is usually deficient in such patients. The drug appears to stimulate hair growth and drying of seborrheic skin. Improvement was noted after treatment of patients with seborrheic alopecia, acne vulgaris and alopecia areata."

In January, 1975, Robert B. Northway, D.V.M., Catheys Valley, CA, in his paper, "Experimental use of Aloe vera Extract in Clinical Practice," published in Veterinary Medicine, reported on the use of Aloe vera to treat ringworm, atopy (allergy), abscess, otisis externa, hot spots, miscellaneous fungal infections, lacerations, lip fold dermatitis, inflamed cyst and staphyloma.

Dr. Northway's subjects included forty-two dogs, twenty-two cats, and four horses. Dr. Northway found that, in all cases, good to excellent results were achieved when Aloe vera was used to treat various skin disorders and/or diseases which affected the test animals. The report does show that in four cases, poor results or no changes were noted. Poor results were mentioned in one case of hot spots and in one case of lip fold dermatitis; no results were achieved in two cases of otitis externa.

Dr. Northway mentioned that the study was completed during a period of one to four weeks, and application was performed by rubbing the Aloe vera onto the lesions one to four times daily.

In the 1980's, Dr. Bill Wolfe, D.D.S., P.A., Albuquerque, NM, in association with Dr. Eugene Zimmerman, and the Baylor College of Dentistry, Dallas, TX, performed the most extensive study ever undertaken on the use of Aloe vera as a treatment for dental-related disorders. The Aloe vera compound used in these studies was yellow in color and had a somewhat bitter taste and odor. The study was designed to test Aloe vera as a significant agent in combating dental disease and promoting healing. The study was divided into a number of categories to determine the efficacy and safety of the product prior to use in patient treatment.

The first part was a bactericidal study performed to determine the level at which various concentrations of Aloe would kill or impede the growth of various organisms including:

Staphylococcus Aureus, Streptococcus Viridaus, Candida Albicans, Corynebacterium Xerosis, and the five strains of Streptococcus Mutant most commonly found in dental plaque. The researchers found that the gel was very bacteriocidal against the above organisms and fungicidal against Candida Albicans (the cause of moniliasis, or "denture sore mouth").

An important finding by Zimmerman was that the dramatic bacterial effects of the Aloe vera was not evident until a 70% concentration was used; to insure control, the Aloe product used was a 90 per cent concentrate. In Virucidal studies, Aloe vera oral gel was found to be virucidal against Herpes virus, a strain of Simplex I, and the strain Zoster.

In Anti-inflammatory studies, Aloe vera was also compared to prednisolone and indomethacin (common anti-inflammatory drugs) which were used in comparative studies with Aloe vera oral gel to observe effects on tissue culture cells. The Aloe gel was found to be just as effective as the Prednisolone and Indomethacin, without having the long term toxicity of either drug.

To determine toxicity, a cell cytotoxicity study was conducted. "Human embryonic kidney cells (HEK) were utilized to determine the effectiveness of Aloe vera on cellular longevity. The cellular death rate was found to be reduced by 2/3 when cultured with the Aloe vera. It was found to be "non-toxic, bacteriocidal, virucidal, fungucidal, an anti-inflammatory agent, a stimulant of cellular life-extension, and have anesthetic effects while it heals."

In a Prosthodontics study, it was shown that Aloe vera was highly effective as a treatment for sore areas in the mouth, as an effective product to be applied under dentures, (See photos, Figures 1, 2, 3, and 4, end of chapter 13), around temporary crowns to eliminate soreness, and to help alleviate irritation and swelling.

Dr. Wolfe recommends that the gel be rubbed around permanent crowns and encourages patients to use Aloe vera on the gingival margins around the crowns by massaging the product into the gums with their fingers. Concerning the periodontic study, Dr.Wolfe states that in "Acute necrotizing ulcerative gingivitis, the objective is to alleviate the symptoms so that a thorough debridement can be performed. The first visit usually consists of a careful, spot scaling or cavitron utilization. After oral hygiene instruction it is stressed to the patient to apply the Aloe vera as often as possible to the infected area, with their finger, interdental stimulator, or irrigation syringe, as indicated by the pocket depths involved."

For endodonitics, Dr. Wolfe indicated that Aloe vera is effective as a lubricant on files. Before inserting into the canals, Dr. Wolfe explained, "I dip the file into a small amount of Aloe vera on a mixing pad. I am not concerned if any of the gel is extruded out the apex, as research has demonstrated Aloe to be non-toxic and regenerative to tissue cells."

Dr. Wolfe also states that Aloe vera is effective as a treatment following oral surgery. He recommended that it be applied to the socket at least three times daily, either with finger tips or a monojet syringe (See photos, Figures 5 and 6, end of chapter 13). The entire socket should be flushed with Aloe vera, and noted that it is so penetrating that many patients experience a temporary anesthesia of the alvolar nerve from such deep penetration.

Wolfe also investigated Temporomandibular joint syndrome. He concluded that the symptoms must be treated first before the syndrome can be managed. Muscle spasms and pain were treated pallatively so that relaxation could be achieved and the causative elements dealt with.

Concluding with a study of Oral Pathology, Dr. Wolfe emphasized that Aloe vera is virucidal, bacteriocidal, and fungicidal. He found that Aloe was an effective treatment for oral lesions involving herpes ulcerations which was a common emesis of the patients studied. Wolfe concluded that Aloe vera gel should be applied to the affected area as often as possible using cotton-tipped applicators or the fingertips.

He also addressed a special note to dental professionals, suggesting that they investigate, experiment and conclude for themselves, the effectiveness, new uses, and exciting future for Aloe vera within dentistry.

As stated earlier, some have credited the plant's vitamins, amino acids, enzymes, simple sugars, or minerals for its ability to heal. Others maintain that Aloe vera gel contains water which is different from the water found in other plants, leaving the false impression that the water in Aloe vera plants possesses some sort of magic properties. While it is true that the value of the gel is in its nutrients, we have also established the fact that the rind and the sap contain many of the same nutrients plus other agents, and in some cases, in much higher amounts. But, we believe these theories do not completely explain the ability of Aloe to heal. Other plausible theories must be investigated while we remember that the gel plays its part.

An interesting and comprehensive theory on the healing

ability of Aloe vera was put forward in a series of three papers by John Heggars, M.D. of the Chicago Burn Center and his colleagues. The papers are: 1. "The Therapeutic Efficacy of Aloe vera Cream in Thermal Injury: Two Case Reports," 2. "Frostbite Injuries: A Rational Approach Based on Pathophysiology" both published in the September/October, 1980, issue of the Journal of American Animal Hospital Association, and 3. "Myth, Magic, Witchcraft, or Fact? Aloe vera Revisited" in the May, 1982 issue of the Journal of Burn Care Rehabilitation. Heggars and his associates not only demonstrate the healing ability of the Aloe but also list the chemical components of the plant which they believe accomplish that healing . (See Tables 1-6, at the end of this chapter).

All this is important for it shows that if papers are to be written on the subject, they should include the chemistry of the substance used if they are to be deemed totally valid. This is true because such information is vital to good research, and without it, we are not sure what part of the plant was used, no matter how good an explanation may be given as to how the plant was processed.

In the studies under discussion, Heggars and his associates attribute the ability of Aloe vera to heal third degree burns and frost bite to the presence in the plant of salicylates (which are broken down by Kolbe's reaction), and the presence of fatty acids such as cholesterol, Triglycerides, and cell membrane phospholipids which are precursors of the arachidonic acid cascade. Heggars notes that Brasher, Zimmermann, and Collings were correct when they stated that Aloe contains prostaglandin inhibitors (anti-inflammatory agents) similar to prednisolone and indometacin, but less toxic to cell cultures than synthetic, man-made prostaglandin inhibitors. (See Table 4, end of this chapter).

The study also confirms the findings of Gottschall and others by explaining that it is the barbaloin in Aloe vera which makes it a highly effective anti-microbial agent. (See Tables 5 and 6, end of this chapter). Heggars states that Aloe in concentrations of 70% to 90% was just as effective as Silver Sulfadiazine (most widely used agent for control of infection in burns and other topical injuries), and he further explains the pain-killing properties of the plant by noting that it contains magnesium and salicylic acid (aspirin-like compound).

He summarizes by saying, "Aloe vera, therefore, has three major properties that are most beneficial in thermal injury: (1) Either due to its aspirin-like effect or the high magnesium content, or probably both acting synergistically, it can potentiate an anesthetic effect; (2) It has a broad spectrum anti-microbial effect, especially against agents responsible for burn wound sepsis; and (3) It has antiprostanoid or, specifically, an anti-thromboxane effect. This latter property may be due to its biochemical configuration which allows the compound to act as an enzomatic substrate competitor.

"Aloe vera has an abundance of fatty acids, which probably supply the necessary nutrients required for normal tissue maturation...Therefore, Aloe inhibits thromboxane production by competitive inhibition through sterochemical means, it also supplies the necessary precursors to initiate the arachidonic cascade giving the cell the important constitutes (PGE and PGF2a) to maintain cell integrity." He concludes by saying, "These experimental data clearly suggest that a 70% concentration extract of Aloe vera can be beneficial in a burn wound."

At the 1983 annual meeting of the National Aloe Science Council, Dr. Heggars presented a summary of these studies. In his final remarks to the NASC, Dr. Heggars specifically stated that the gel of the plant was not responsible for the results he had achieved; it was the anthraquinone glucosides (sap), and within these final comments, he specifically stated that the only thing that really matters was the fact that Aloe vera is an effective treatment for burns -- it works.

The chemistry of Aloe included in Heggars' 1982 paper is fully substantiated by an earlier report, a 1978 paper published by Oklahoma State University, which also states that Aloe contains cholesterol and triglycerides (fatty acids), but unlike the Chicago paper, identifies two of these fatty acids specifically as campesterol and b-sitosterol.

The OSU study also identifies another source of Aloe's anti-microbial and pain-killing effects by confirming the presence of Lupeol, a hydrochloride, in the juice of the leaf. But unlike the Russian study mentioned, neither OSU nor Heggars mentions the presence of urea nitrogen and cinnammonic acid.

In a 1987 article published in the magazine, Woman's World, Dr. Rosalie Burns, M.D., a professor and chairman of the Department of Neurology, The Medical College of Pennsylvania, Philadelphia, PA, discusses the effect of Aloe vera on shingles in the article titled, "Shingles--One Rash, Three Problems." Dr. Burns identifies and describes the disease commonly known as shingles (Herpes Zoster).

She points out that shingles is caused by the same virus that also causes chicken pox and common herpes of the mouth and sexual organs. "The strange virus doesn't disappear after the child recovers (from Chicken Pox), she writes. Instead, it remains in the body, lying dormant in the spinal nerves for many years--often forever -- inactive and harmless. But sometimes, for reasons that aren't clearly understood, the virus is reactivated. When that happens, it reappears -- this time as shingles."

"As shingles, the virus travels along the sensory nerves to the skin, causing a rash of blisters, usually on the trunk or face, triggering intense pain and itching and posing the threat of a severe secondary infection."

Of interest to us is the fact that the doctor concludes her article by stating, "Sap from the leaves of the Aloe vera plant is an old folk remedy that relieves pain and speeds healing when spread over the blisters."

This article suggests that Gottshall was onto something important when he reported that Aloe vera sap was a highly effective killing agent for the Tuberculosis Baccilis, the same virus discussed by Dr. Burns.

History and medical studies teach that it is the sap (anthraquinone glucoside) which contains the plant's healing and anti-inflammatory agents, and it is the gel which is responsible for its ability to penetrate the skin. However, if this were not enough to convince the skeptic that the healing agents are located in the sap not in the gel, then the skeptic has nowhere else to turn but to his belief in myth and magic...for that is how the gel has always been promoted.

AIDS--A New Frontier In Research

Since 1987, it has apparently been relatively common knowledge among AIDS victims in the Dallas-Fort Worth area that Aloe juice or a drug (Polymannoacetate) derived from it will provide relief from the symptoms of the disease and will keep those who have the virus but who do not have any of the symptoms of AIDS from developing the disease.

Even though the evidence available is preliminary, we feel that because the work was done at the Dallas-Ft.Worth Medical Center, Grand Prairie, Texas and because of the status of the physicians involved, the work is important, and we believe we would be remiss in not reporting the results achieved thus far.

It is very important to understand that this research does not show that Aloe vera is a cure for AIDS, but it does indicate that in all cases examined, excellent results were achieved and that in a majority of test cases, Aloe vera stopped the progress of the disease. In other words, Aloe is not a cure for AIDS but is a highly effective treatment.

This premise was first put forward in an article "Aloe Drug May Mimic AZT Without Toxicity," in Medical World News, December, 1987. The article reported on the research work of Dr. H. Reg McDaniel. According to Dr. McDaniel, "A substance in the Aloe plant shows preliminary signs of boosting AIDS patients' immune systems and blocking the human immune-deficiency virus' spread without toxic side effects."

The results of Dr. McDaniel's pilot study showed that the symptoms of sixteen 16 AIDS patients were significantly reduced when given 1,000 mg a day of the drug for three months. After three months, six patients with advanced cases of AIDS showed a 20 per cent improvement in symptoms, while less seriously ill patients improved by an average of 71 per cent. Dr. McDaniel has also reported his research findings at the combined meeting of the American Society of Clinical Pathologists and College of American Pathologists.

He says, "Fever and symptoms of night sweats, diarrhea, and opportunistic infections were either eliminated or significantly improved in all patients, with corresponding drops in HIV antibody positive cell cultures and HIV core antigen levels."

Red cell mass increased in all but one patient, and twelve initially leukopeic patients had a slight rise in white count after treatment.

No toxic effects have been noted in a total of twenty-nine patients who have now received the experimental drug.

There is also evidence that good quality Aloe vera juice can relieve the symptoms of AIDS. This is not surprising since the drug (Polymannoacetate) is produced by the plant and would be present in the juice.

An article by Irwin Frank in the Tuesday, July 12, 1988 edition of The Dallas Times Herald quotes Dr. Terry Pulse as saying that 20 ounces of Aloe vera juice, with the drug stabilized in the Aloe, was administered orally to 69 AIDS patients." (Apparently, the doctor means stabilized Aloe vera juice.)

According to the article, Pulse says the patients treated with the drug were classified as those who would "never improve or get better," but following treatment, were able to "return to normal work". The article quoted Pulse as saying that these patients "go back to their standard energy level, their symptoms disappear almost completely -- and that's in 81 per cent of the patients that I put on this drug."

He adds that those patients with the AIDS virus who showed no symptoms of the disease remained free of symptoms while taking the drug which is derived from the Aloe vera plant.

"The sooner you can get a patient on this drug, the better off they are," says Pulse. He said his patients take 20 ounces of the liquid a day, "and I keep them on it indefinitely. I've had some of them on it for over two years."

"We have had deaths," he says, "but in those patients (who died), most can be attributed to having gone and gotten chemotherapy for skin cancers, or whatever, or have taken other drugs in combination that knocked out their immune system, such as AZT."

When asked what his study and treatment meant as far as an AIDS treatment or cure is concerned, Pulse replied, "It means that until there is a magic bullet, this is a stopgap measure and it buys them (the AIDS patients) time at a fraction of the cost" of AZT.

After reading this article, we obtained copies of the actual research data published by Dr. Pulse together with his colleagues, H. R. McDaniel and T. Reg Watson, all of the Dallas-Ft. Worth Medical Center. This information was evaluated to eliminate the confusing aspects concerning exactly what was used in the study, whether the product was Aloe vera juice or the drug or both and in what percentages.

From this data and further investigation, it appears that

Aloe vera juice in its natural state is just as effective a treatment for AIDS as the freeze dried drug derived from it. It is obvious that any AIDS patient who believes that Aloe vera might help his condition should be very careful to buy only real 100% Aloe vera juice which, as we have noted repeatedly, neither looks nor tastes like water. Real Aloe, we repeat, is amber colored and has a rather bitter taste.

Shown below are the tables from Myth, magic, witchcraft, or fact? Aloe vera revisited. *Journal of Burn Care and Rehabilitation* 3, 157-163. Robson, M.C., Heggers, J.P. and Hagstrom, W.J. (1982). University of Chicago Burn Center, Chicago.

Table 1.- Biochemical Constituents of *Aloe vera* Extract Determined by SMAC

Constituent	Quantity
Glucose	13 mg/dl
Uric acid	0.5 mg/dl
Salicylic acid	3.6 mg/dl
Creatinine	1.9 mg/dl
Alkaline phosphatase	1 IU/L
Creatine phosphokinase	10 IU/L
Cholesterol	11 mg/dl
Triglycerides	374 mg/dl
Lactate	14.8 mg/dl
Total protein	0.2 mg/dl

Table 2. - Inorganic Constituents of *Aloe vera* Extract

Constituent	Quantity
Sodium	19.0 mEq/L
Potassium	21.5 mEq/L
Inorganic phosphorus	14.0 mg/dl
Chloride	1.0 mEq/L

Table 3. - Trace metal analysis of *Aloe vera* Extract

Constituent	Quantity
Calcium	23.5 mEq/L
Magnesium	4.6 mg/dL
Copper	0.2 mg/dL
Zinc	0.02 mg/dL

Table 4. - Antimicrobial Effects of Aloe vera Extract in Cream Base compared to Silver Sulfadiazine in Agar Well Diffusion (Zone Sizes Measured in mm

Organisms	Aloe vera	AgSD
Gram negative		
E. Coli	16	12
Enterobacter cloacae	14	12
K. pneumoniae	14	6*
P. aeruginosa	17	12
Gram positive		
S. aureus	18	12
S. pyogenes	16	12
S. agalatiae	16	12
S. faecalis	6	11
B. subtilis	19	14

*Agar well is 6mm in diameter.

Table 5. - Immunohistochemical Analysis of Aloe and Methimazole Treated Tissue Compared with Untreated Burn Tissue

Prostanoid derivative	Aloe vera (Time [hr])			Methimazole (Time [hr])			Control (Time [hr])		
	8	24	72	8	24	72	8	24	72
PGE2	3+	4+	3+	4+	4+	3+	2+	2+	1+
PGF2a	2+	2+	2+	2+	1+	1+	3+	4+	3+
TxB2	0	0	0	1+	0	0	3+	4+	3+
Normal rabbit serum control	0	0	0	0	0	0	0	0	0

Table 6. - Antimicrobial Effects of *Aloe vera* Extract (CFU/ml/conc. of extract)

Organisms	100%	90%	80%	70%	60%
Gram negative					
E. coli	≤4	≤4	≤4	2.4X10₃	8.0X10₄
Citrobacter sp.	≤4	≤4	≤4	≤4	≤4
S. marcescens	≤4	≤4	≤4	≤4	≤4
Enterobacter sp.	≤4	≤4	≤4	≤4	20
Klebsiella sp.	≤4	≤4	≤4	≤4	≤4
P. aeruginosa	≤4	≤4	≤4	≤4	12
Gram positive					
S. aureus	≤4	≤4	≤4	≤4	1.5X10₂
S. pyogenes, group A	≤4	≤4	≤4	28	40
S. agalactiae, group B	≤4	≤4	≤4	≤4	≤4
S. sp., group D	≤4	≤4	10₄-10₅	5.5X10₆	7.2X10₆
B. subtilis	2.2X10₄	2.5X10₄	2.2X10₄	1.9X10₄	2.8X10₄
Yeast					
C. albicans	≤4	≤4	≤10₃	2.9X10₃	2.7X10₆

CHAPTER ELEVEN

ECONOMICS OF ALOE VERA

This Economics of Aloe vera chapter will, we hope, serve as a guide to help you develop a common sense approach to growing, processing marketing, buying, and drinking Aloe vera juice and using cosmetics made with or containing Aloe vera. We hope this section will help you to judge the difference between the claims made and the product delivered.

There is a myth that the Aloe vera plant has no medical value until it has large leaves (over one pound) and is from two to four years of age, an idea which is disproved by the fact that even plants with small leaves (3 to 4 ounces) and grown on the windowsill, have outstanding benefits. On the other hand, it does take the young plant (or pup), which grows from the root of the mother-plant, a few weeks to begin producing the sap; this explains why household pets, especially cats, will eat the pup for a short period after it appears. It is not the age of the plant which explains its medical value; still, large leaves are critical to the success of the commercial grower.

Some "authorities" state that Aloe vera grows best in poor soil, requires a minimum of water, and requires no fertilizer. This simply is not so. Even though the plant will survive under such conditions, it will not thrive and produce large leaves of commercial value as quickly. Probably such erroneous ideas exist because some have incorrectly identified Aloe vera as a cactus, and in so doing, have come to the false conclusion that it is a desert plant. Aloe vera is a tropical plant which will survive and even thrive in the wettest of environments.

Growing Aloe vera for Fun

Under ideal growing conditions, usable leaves can be produced from small pups in sixteen to eighteen months, but two years is more realistic because it is almost impossible to create ideal growing conditions unless the plants are grown in greenhouses, and even then it is difficult.

If grown under poor conditions, the plant may never produce leaves of commercial size. Most Aloe vera plants growing on windowsills or in small pots will never flower. The plant will remain small, but even these small plants will reproduce themselves by pupping.

The Aloe vera plant is fun to grow. It can be a beautiful flowering addition to your house or office, a most welcome guest, and a conversation piece--your own first-aid kit in a pot.

Grow the plant in increasingly large pots of loose, sandy soil with adequate drainage (never allow the plant to stand in water -- or to become too dry). Feed with a water-soluble houseplant or vegetable fertilizer. Water the plant as often as necessary and feed as directed. Give adequate, but not direct, sunlight. The plant grows best in a large window or a sun-room where the air temperature is between 75 degrees and 85 degrees Fahrenheit.

Growing Aloe vera for Profit

Under normal growing conditions, a field-grown Aloe vera plant with leaves weighing from one to one and one-half pounds, yields two and one-half to five gallons of liquid per year when the plant is cut twice a year. Each plant requires at least six square feet of growing space, but bigger and healthier plants can be produced if nine square feet is allotted per plant. A one-acre field of Aloe vera can contain as many as 8,000 or so plants, but 5,400 to 6,000 is a more realistic figure.

Anyone interested in growing Aloe vera commercially has very important facts to consider, for the commercial viability of any such project is critical. The land used to grow Aloe vera is generally very expensive when compared to the normal cost of cropland in the United States. The growing site must be in a region where temperatures do not fall to freezing or below. In the United States, such regions include the Rio Grande Valley of Texas, Southern California, and Florida.

This land must be in an area where the fields can be irrigated properly without allowing the plants to stand in water which will drown the plants. It must be of a sandy loam and, ideally, should be slightly sloped because this encourages drainage. Furthermore, the soil must be close to the proper Ph, and the cost of bringing the soil to the proper Ph may be prohibitive. Lastly, don't forget the cost of fertilizer to sustain a healthy crop. There must be an ample supply of water low in sodium content.

Aloe acreage will be tied up for at least two years before the first harvest. Start-up costs, and the costs of long-term cultivation must be considered. Both cultivation and harvesting of the plant are expensive processes because both must be done mostly by hand, especially harvesting...A minimum of three full- time workers (or more) are required to take care of one acre of Aloe vera. The workers must weed, cultivate, irrigate, fertilize, remove young pups from the mother plants, and regularly monitor the plants' progress and health. As many as eight to ten additional workers may be required to harvest the leaves.

While it is true that Aloe vera is one crop where insecticides and pesticides would not normally be necessary for the control of insects or pests, there are organisms which will attack the Aloe vera plant. Research shows that this will normally occur only if plants are unhealthy. One organism that will attack the root of the Aloe vera plant, healthy or otherwise, is tobacco fungus. Luckily this problem is easy to control by simply keeping tobacco products out of the growing area...i.e. no smoking, no chewing, no dipping -- no tobacco products of any kind...cigarettes, pipe tobaccos, snuff or chewing tobacco.

Aphids, various forms of rust, weevils, beetles, or other insects can also attack the plants. Generally, this period of susceptibility only occurs when the Aloe vera plants are flowering or are unhealthy.

It is necessary to monitor the crop closely when the plant is flowering because, during this period, the sap is absorbed from the leaves. At such times, most of the sap disappears from the plant. The vulnerability of the plant, especially to insects, can be directly attributed to the movement of the sap (anthraquinone glycosides) from the leaves of the plant to the stem and flower. Somehow the ancients discovered this fact and harvested just before flowering. As Pliny the Elder put it, harvest the sap just before the Rising of the Dog Star.

Another major investment required for Aloe production is for equipment to harvest the crop. This requires large trailers in which to move the leaves from the field to the processing plant (or to an area to be boxed, if a third party is to process the leaves.)

If the grower chooses to process the crop himself, an additional investment of at least $75,000 is required to build a processing facility. Such a facility or processing plant requires the following equipment: leaf washers, filet machine to extract the juice from the leaf, processing kettles in which to heat and stabilize the juice, and pumps and filters to produce a usable juice for beverage or cosmetic products. All of these processing steps can be accomplished by hand, but this could double, or possibly triple the cost per gallon, depending on labor costs.

Under ideal outdoor conditions, each plant will produce from 25 to 50 pounds of leaf per year the lower number if the plant is cut once, and the higher number if the plant is cut twice a year. If the 50 pound figure is achieved, then one acre will produce approximately 120,000 pounds of leaf per year, yielding approximately one gallon of juice per ten pounds of Aloe leaves or approximately 12,000 gallons of juice per acre. Reasonable production figures would be 20-25 per cent less than these maximum numbers. Therefore, on average, one could expect to gross around $60,000 per acre, give or take a few thousand dollars. Return on investment could be much lower, depending on weather conditions, water quality, fertilizer costs, labor, and the price of raw Aloe vera juice at the time of sale.

Currently, the value of raw Aloe vera juice is $4.50 to $5.50 per gallon if purchased in wholesale lots of between 1,000 and 5,000 gallons. Retail packaging of the product could require an investment of between $10,000 and $100,000 (or more) depending on how sophisticated a system is required. Realistically, one could expect to receive between $7.50 and $8.00 per gallon for the finished product. .

Needless to say, anyone who is considering growing Aloe vera commercially must be prepared to invest a tremendous amount of capital in the venture. Quality land suitable for Aloe cultivation is worth $1,000 an acre or more. The land will be tied up in a single crop for at least two years before yielding its first harvest. And don't forget that such land could be used for growing other vegetables which could be harvested quicker and more often and could produce more income more quickly.

Obviously, anyone considering Aloe vera as a commercial venture must be willing to make a long-term investment in equipment, land, capital, labor, time, and energy. While the rewards can be substantial, the risks are great, especially if the product is grown in a place where occasional freezes occur. One freeze can wipe out years of investment as the growers of the Rio Grande Valley sadly learned several years ago.

Bottom Line

Currently, the wholesale price of processed 100% Aloe

vera juice varies from $4.50 to $5.50 per gallon. Approximately one-half (or less) of these dollars goes to the grower who sells leaf to be processed by others. The wholesale price of leaf is 15 to 25 cents a pound. Ten pounds of leaf produces up to one gallon of juice. Therefore, the grower can expect a gross return of between $1.50 to $2.50 per 10 pounds of leaf produced. Assuming the price of raw juice averages $5.00 per gallon, the processor may gross up to $3.50 per gallon, but $2.50 is more realistic.

If the grower, processor, and packager are one and the same, the finished 100% (meaning no water added) juice can cost as much as $7.50 or more per gallon, but don't forget the cost of containers, plastic or glass, costing from 35 cents to 50 cents per unit, plus caps, seals and label costs, all of which can cost from 40 to 60 cents per container. Add in the cost of shipping cartons, handling, and shipping costs. And, if that were not enough the costs of storing the raw and/or finished product when necessary must obviously be added to the total costs.

Assume the packager wishes to sell 100% Aloe vera juice to a major wholesale/retail outlet which plans to move the product at a retail price of $6.00 to $7.00 per gallon. The obvious question is--based on what you know about the economics of Aloe vera--is it possible to retail 100% Aloe at the price of $6.00 to $7.00 per gallon? Considering that the retailer normally marks up products 35% to 50% and that shipping must be added on (which would then make the wholesale price at least $9.00 to $9.50 per gallon) ask yourself, " is it possible for a grower-processor to sell REAL 100% ALOE VERA JUICE to the retailer for $4.00 or less and make a profit ?" Since few in business will (or can) do something for nothing, and since the costs of growing, processing, and bottling pure 100 % aloe vera are as stated, it is apparent that even a major retailer cannot sell 100% juice for less than $12.00 or more per gallon. If the retailer markets the product at 35% profit, and the product costs $9.00 per gallon including shipping, it must be retailed for at least $12.00. Realistically, most retailers want a 50% mark-up, meaning a 100% product would retail at about $15.00 or more per gallon, minimum. This is assuming that the grower, processor, packager, and broker are one and the same. If not, add on from 10% to 20%. Under these circumstances $16.50 to $19.95 is a realistic price to expect to pay for 100% Aloe vera. However, these prices are based on maximum productivity and are, therefore, somewhat unrealistic. In reality 100% Aloe would probably need to sell at retail from between $24.95 to $29.95 per gallon. If you want the product delivered to your door by your friendly and helpful neighborhood direct salesperson, you might reasonably expect to pay $39.95 (or even more) for the real thing.

The answer to the above question is obviously "no" if the product is truly 100% Aloe vera. While it is certainly possible to sell lesser concentrations at a retail price of between $6.00 and $7.00 per gallon, it is impossible to profitably sell 100% Aloe vera for such a retail price. The truth is, the only product which would be inexpensive enough to retail at such prices is a product that has been watered down, and that is exactly what is being sold in many stores, according to laboratory tests made on samples taken at random. Remember, if it looks like water, tastes like water, and smells like water...then there is a good chance that it is water, or that the product contains less than 25% real Aloe or less Aloe vera gel and no sap. And if the product has no color and no taste, it has no medical value.

Therefore, the question becomes is the consumer being cheated? The answer is "no" -- if the product contains enough Aloe to justify the price. A product retailing for $6.00 to $7.00 per gallon should contain between 20% and 30% Aloe vera. As such, it would be no less a bargain than truly 100 per cent Aloe vera. But don't forget, if it ain't "yello or reddo," it ain't Aloe.

If the thought has crossed your mind that you would be interested in using or even growing Aloe vera commercially, then our purpose here has been accomplished, and this information should be of vital interest to you.

CHAPTER TWELVE

ALOE VERA AND COSMETICS

A Natural Approach to Looking Good

Humans have been interested in cosmetics and personal adornment for thousands of years. Today the cosmetics business is a multi-billion dollar a year industry in the United States alone.

Most of the research on Aloe vera in treatment products has been on the plant's therapeutic effect on skin diseases, disorders, and injury. As the Chicago Burn Center Report of 1982 puts it, "The results in the treatment of burn patients attributed to Aloe vera are so miraculous as to seem more like myth than fact."

During the last thirty years, many have used such statements to promote Aloe vera in cosmetics. Today the use of the name to add mystique to cosmetic products has reached an all-time high, with some major brands and thousands of smaller companies offering such products. But like the promoters of Aloe vera as a health drink, many in the cosmetic industry have also played a tune of myth and magic.

According to the article, "Current Status of Aloe As A Cure All" by Gunnar Gjerstad and T. D. Riner (published in the American Journal of Pharmacy, Volume 140, 1968), one cosmetic company ran an advertisement in a major magazine which perfectly illustrates the sales pitch. "If Mother Nature can keep a plant blooming in the deserts, why can't she do the same for a woman's skin? She can (!) -- This organization uses one of Mother Nature's own beauty ingredients, Aloe vera gel, in a new line of skin care products...This precious gel is extracted from the heart of the leaf of the Aloe vera plant. The gel moisturizes and brings the plant to flower and keeps it supple and soft even in intense desert heat. Imagine how moist it can keep a woman's skin."

In reviewing this ad, Gjerstad and Riner said, "Such asinine advertising ought to be prohibited by law; because there are people who will believe that a woman's skin is identical to Aloe jelly."

Unfortunately, such advertisers and authors both misrepresent the truth. The advertiser promotes the idea that the gel is a wonderful moisturizing agent. In fact, moisturizing agents must contain a balance of both oil and water to be truly effective. The ad infers that Aloe gel contains such a balance when, in fact, the oil of the plant is confined to the sap and the rind with none being present in the gel. The authors make a valid criticism, but their points are based on incomplete knowledge. Obviously, the authors do not understand the chemistry of Aloe vera. We have already seen that Aloe vera contains a broad spectrum of agents which are very similar to the chemistry of human skin, although not identical.

The advertiser also infers that it is the gel which keeps the plant soft and supple "in the desert." This is totally fictious. It is water which plays a critical role in keeping the plant alive during drought , and it is the rind and the sap which help keep the plant "supple." But, under extended drought, even these mechanisms fail, and the leaf becomes hard and brittle.

In recent years, another major cosmetics company has chosen not to use Aloe vera "gel" because the company states that their research shows it is not a moisturizer but is, in fact, a drying agent. This writer concurs in that judgement because the gel contains no oil, and without the oil from the sap and/or the rind, Aloe vera is not a moisturizer.

With the above information, one could conclude that the oil produced by the plant is necessary if Aloe vera is used as a moisturizing ingredient in cosmetics. As in the use of Aloe vera as a beverage, there are no standards for its use in cosmetics other than the FDA 50 parts per million limit on sap in any product, regardless of how it is to be used. Consequently, the consumer has no standard by which to judge. He must rely only on the integrity of the manufacturer. But here also, we find through chemical analysis that certain products leave much to be desired. Some purported Aloe products show no traceable amounts of Aloe present, despite the bold use of the name on the package.

Perhaps it is worthwhile to examine the definition of cosmetics so we can come to some logical conclusion as to how Aloe vera can best be utilized in this field. Webster defines cosmetics as "of" or "relating to or making for beauty, especially of the complexion."

Cosmetics, according to the World Book Encyclopedia, are "all substances, preparations, devices and treatments used to cleanse, to alter the appearance, or to promote the attractiveness of the face and body. The use of cosmetics is recorded in the Bible where the practice of anointing the head or body with oils is mentioned. The word comes from the Greek kosmetikos, meaning skilled in decorating.

Among the ancient Egyptians, cosmetics were prepared by physicians. The most famous figure associated with cosmetics was the last queen of Egypt, Cleopatra (69-30 B.C.), who was noted for her skill in making and using cosmetics.

Physicians supplied cosmetics to the Greeks, then to the Romans, the Arabs, and the peoples of Western Europe. Each group added something to the art of cosmetics. Finally, the physicians got too busy to practice the art of adornment.

Cosmetics of the present day include beauty products for the hair, scalp, body, face, and hands. Soap and perfume are related to cosmetics, and so are dentifrices, deodorants, and the hair-removing preparations called depilatories."

The FDA defines cosmetics as, "any article intended to be rubbed, sprinkled, or sprayed on the body or any parts thereof, or introduced into or otherwise applied for the purpose of cleansing, beautifying, promoting attractiveness or altering the appearance, and articles intended for use as components thereof."

In a very real sense the cosmetics industry and the consumer are at a crossroads. Are "cosmetic" products to continue as defined by FDA, or will modern technology and scientific discoveries be allowed to make cosmetics into something which can do much more? Ironically, this movement may bring us full circle, for if the ancient definition is correct, it would appear that products containing Aloe vera (and other natural agents) were used not only for adornment, but also as healing agents.

For example, the Papyrus Ebers says that Aloe was used for the adornment of both men and women, thus referring to both internal and external use to enhance beauty and health, both within and without. Adornment in ancient times was held to mean that health and beauty go hand in hand.

Aloe vera -- The Perfect Ingredient?

Aloe vera is a wonderful cosmetic ingredient, but it is necessary for the manufacturer to understand what Aloe vera is and how to use it. The manufacturer also must have integrity as his ultimate barometer in creating products which deliver what they promise. It is not enough to simply put Aloe vera in the product; indeed it is critical that the formulator understand how much Aloe is necessary in any given product to perform its intended purpose. Given the cost of top quality Aloe vera, logic indicates that putting too much in a product (more than is necessary for its intended purpose) is a waste of the consumer's money.

History, science, and chemistry indicate that the percentage of Aloe vera in a product be determined on the base of its intended purpose. Despite this fact, cosmetics manufacturers who have chosen to use Aloe play an advertising numbers game with each new product, claiming it is the best simply because it contains more Aloe vera than its predecessors. If one claims his product contains 50 per cent, a good marketer will claim his contains 51 per cent, inferring that the 51% product is better. This ploy was pointed out by Albert Leung, Ph.D., in a September, 1985, article in Drug and Cosmetics Industry titled, "Aloe vera Update: A New Form Questions Integrity of Old." Leung asserted that, despite heavy promotion in Aloe vera products, several difficulties still remain including a lack of meaningful identification and purity standards. As a result it is impossible to mount a successful challenge to producer claims that they have the best or purest products.

He further states that the notion that even trace amounts of aloin in the gel render it ineffective and even harmful is untrue. This erroneous belief has prompted Aloe vera suppliers to stress the low aloin content of their gels (even though it is common knowledge to those who have used Aloe vera gel from freshly split leaves that fresh gels always contain certain levels of the bitter yellow juice (aloin), without loss of efficacy.

Leung's article drew comments in two letters, published in the December, 1985, <u>Drug and Cosmetics.</u> The first, authored by R. C. Benson of Harlingen, TX, stated, "I have allowed some time to pass after reading the article by Dr. Leung in the September issue, so that I might give considerable thought to an answer. What was so frustrating in reading the article was that it was just another article dealing with whose Aloe or what type Aloe is best. That might have been the issue three or four years ago, but I don't believe it is today. Frankly, I don't think a majority of major health and beauty aid products companies care which is best. Their primary interest is price and they want to be able to put Aloe on the front label panel as inexpensively as possible (since there are no standards to challenge at present). Thus, it is the consumer who loses, since he or she pays a higher price for a perceived added value that is not being realized.

The sad part about all this is that Aloe is a wonderful ingredient that does so many positive things. Many consumers have tried to experience this but have been frustrated by the products they have purchased," he added.

"DCI has been the leader in publishing articles on Aloe and we appreciate that. While it may not be always possible, maybe I expect such a fine publication to present only the side of the just and the correct!," Benson concluded.

The second letter, authored by Elliott Farber, of Fargo, North Dakota, stated that the article, "spends three pages stating there are no analytical methods that can really establish the activity or concentration of commercial grades of Aloe vera gel."

Further, Farber states in his letter that the article under review is nothing more than an article to promote one company's process over another. Lunge's article refers to a specific Aloe vera processor which he claims "produces a natural, genuine dehydrated Aloe vera gel.

"The question," writes Farber, " that comes to my mind, (as I am sure it must have come to that of Dr. Leung at some time) is that if there are no current analytical methods to ascertain Aloe vera gel purity, how can one demonstrate in an acceptable scientific manner that when reconstituted, one Aloe vera product is better than another."

He concluded by stating, "The format of the article in questioning the veracity of competitive Aloe vera products, then lauding another without the proof required of the original version is a poor example for anyone to set."

It is fascinating to note that Dr. Leung responded to these letters, "Since only fresh Aloe vera gel is well known for its consistently beneficial properties and since its active components remain unknown, the less we subject the gel to processing, the more active the processed gel is likely to be..."

It is apparent that Dr. Leung was not aware of the work done by the National Aloe Science Council which is referred to by Benson in his letter, nor was he aware of the vast number of chemical analyses which have been performed. As a final minor point, aloin is not the bitter sap of the leaf, as mistakenly asserted by Dr. Leung. And although it is a minor point technically, it is a major point chemically.

Today, the Aloe vera industry can be compared to a number of small children fighting in the playground over who has the biggest, the best, and the most.

And, as Benson writes, the loser here is the consumer. The use of Aloe vera as a cosmetic ingredient is at the same point where standards must be established and adhered to.

CHAPTER THIRTEEN

SEEING IS BELIEVING!

The old phrase, "Seeing is believing," applies perfectly to my personal experience with Aloe vera. I was born with a wide range of severe allergies which, frankly, made life very unpleasant for many years. In 1968, I was seen at the Oklahoma Allergy Clinic where I was tested for allergic reaction to some 180 separate substances. The testing revealed that I was allergic to 178 of the substances and highly allergic to 150 of them. In addition, I had large patches of severe atopic dermatitis on the inside of both arms at the elbows and the back of both knees, on the scalp, armpits, neck, ankles, and groin; I continually suffered from itchy watery eyes and sinus congestion and infections caused by the allergies. After diagnosis I began a battery of injections for my problem. They did not improve my condition.

I was also seen by one of the most respected dermatologists in the Oklahoma City area. She prescribed ultraviolet light treatments and a coal-tar based ointment (which has since been banned as unsafe).. Both provided only a small amount of relief.

Not until I learned about and began experimenting with Aloe vera in 1973 did I get some relief for my skin problems by using an Aloe based "jelly" product which was a combination of sap and gel. Unfortunately, I did not then have any knowledge that Aloe could be used for drinking, for I still believed the prevailing nonsense which claimed that the sap was poison. Not until six years ago, when I seriously began to study both the historical and scientific evidence concerning the plant, did I begin to drink top-quality 100% Aloe vera. I knew it was real Aloe because I processed it myself. To my amazement and delight, my allergies completely disappeared shortly after I began to drink Aloe daily. I then noticed that if I did not regularly consume Aloe, my allergies returned, so I began to experiment. Between January and June of 1984, I went off and on Aloe drink in regular two week cycles. I discovered that when I drank the product every day, my allergies disappeared, and when I ceased to drink Aloe, my allergies came right back.

Although I had not completed my investigation to discover why Aloe worked, I had personally experienced its benefits and since I definitely didn't want the allergies back, I began drinking Aloe everyday, and I continue to drink it as of this writing. Today, I have no apparent allergies but know from experience that if I stop drinking Aloe, the symptoms will return. In addition, my lifelong atopic dermatitis has disappeared completely. But Aloe has done more than help my allergies.

By drinking Aloe every day, I have completely eliminated the chronic indigestion from which I suffered along with constipation and kidney infection. I am now completely free of hemorrhoids due, I believe, to systematic applications of concentrated Aloe ointment and more regular digestion and elimination. I have cut my cholesterol level in half, although I must attribute that result somewhat to a change in diet. I also believe that drinking Aloe has stopped the pain and slowed down the development of arthritis in my knees and ankles due to sports injuries for which I underwent four major surgeries as a teenager and young adult. I do know that when I began drinking Aloe, my legs quit hurting, and the pain does not return as long as I remember to drink the juice daily.

Aloe has increased my energy level, and I might add that during the last five years I have not had a severe cold, the flu, or any type of major internal infection while many of my friends have repeatedly suffered such problems. I could go on, but I think you get the point.

My belief in Aloe vera is much deeper than my knowledge of its history, chemistry, and the medical reports I have studied. It is obviously based on personal experience and, I must also say, tempered by the knowledge that there are medical problems the plant does not benefit! Because I am an Aloe vera grower and processor, some may jump to the conclusion that I have an economic interest in the public and scientific acceptance of Aloe vera. As a matter of fact, I do. But the fact that an individual has an economic interest does not automatically mean that he is an untrustworthy reporter of facts. To repeat, I became interested in Aloe because of what it did for me and what I have seen it do for others. My economic involvement with Aloe grew from my deep interest in spreading the word about what real top-quality Aloe vera can do, not vice versa.

One is seldom allowed to dramatically see the results of his work as it affects the lives of others. The following is a mere sample of what I have seen Aloe vera do for people, many of whom had exhausted orthodox medical advice without much relief.

Odus M. Hennessee

What I have seen Aloe vera do.

On March 17, 1985, a 60 year old man, Reverend Alfed Thompson, came to see me. Thompson stated that both of his legs had been burned in a terrible fire in 1953. Thompson had been horribly burned when a can of gasoline exploded in his hand, drenching him with burning fuel. Thompson was so badly burned that he continually developed a large number of ulcers that would not respond to any treatment other than skin grafts. When asked the number of skin grafts he had received, Thompson said that he had stopped counting after 22. He mentioned that his doctors had told him that the ulcers were due to thin scar tissue and poor circulation. He added that he had also been told that the ulcer would not heal because of the poor circulation.

At the time Thompson had a large ulcer, which was about two months old, on his leg. He said that his doctor had been treating the place for about a month. He went on to say that his leg hurt so much that he could not sleep at night, despite taking 4 to 5 tablets of Acetaminophen each day. He was also applying Neosporin ointment (as prescribed by his physician) four or five times daily. He said that the doctor had told him that the ulcer was clean and ready to be skin grafted. When asked if additional therapy was used, Thompson said that he was picking the dead skin out of the ulcer daily, and once a week the doctor removed dead skin after whirlpool therapy.

The ulcer was located on the outside half of the right leg approximately six inches above the ankle. The ulcer was very light pink (almost white), approximately one inch wide, nearly two inches high, and approximately one quarter inch deep. (See photos , Figures 7, 8, 9, and 10, end of this chapter).

Between March 17 and April 2, Thompson treated the ulcer himself in the following manner. The ulcer was soaked for fifteen minutes in a bath of betadine solution after which three percent hydrogen peroxide was applied. The ulcer was flushed with tap water and a thick layer (enough to completely fill the ulcer) of concentrated Aloe vera ointment (in a base of USP petrolatum) was applied.

On April 2, the daily soaking was discontinued while continuing the application of Aloe ointment. Between April 2 and May 14, no bandages were used when Thompson was relaxing because it was found that the thick layer of ointment provided ample protection from reinfection. However, bandages were used when he was working or sleeping. Thompson said that (due to the Aloe ointment) the pain was reduced greatly and after about two weeks, because of the Aloe ointment, it was generally eliminated. By May 14, 1985, the ulcer was completely healed, with minimal or no scar tissue and approximately fifty percent of the new tissue was normally pigmented. When last seen in 1987, this ulcer was completely healed, 90% normally pigmented, and no apparent breakdown had occurred. To confirm this fact, a dermatologist (who, incidentally, asked to remain anonymous) examined Thompson at my request. The doctor not only stated that the ulcer was free of scar tissue and completely healed, but added that the area had been regenerated. According to the doctor, the skin not only was completely healed but looked like new skin which had never been burned.

Please take particular note that in the above description, we indicate that Reverend Thompson remained under his doctor's care during his course of home treatment with Aloe ointment and that a second physician saw him to confirm that the ulcer was healed. It seems to us that it is very foolish not to take advantage of modern medical care. On the other hand, it is also worth pointing out that the patient's body belongs entirely to the patient and not to the physician. The simple truth is that in the past, patients have tended to be remarkably deferential to physicians.

Obviously, the trained physician is the first authority who should be consulted in the case of illness or injury. But what if, after years of treatment, the sufferer remains in substantially the same condition with little or no improvement for their life-altering condition? It seems obvious to us that in such a situation, the individual has a sovereign right to seek relief in alternative methods.

Aloe vera has long been famous for its effect on burns. It is impossible to accurately estimate the number of Aloe plants sitting on windowsills across America for the express purpose of sacrificing a fat, juicy leaf when a member of the family carelessly burns his hand or scrapes a knee. It is equally futile for the powers-that-be to try to tell the Moms of America that Aloe vera is useless for household burns and scrapes. Mom has used the same darned plant over and over. It works! And it works quick!

Several years ago I received a letter from Mr. Johnny P. Howard who described what Aloe vera had done for his badly burned foot, and he described it as "miraculous." (See photos, Figures 11, 12, 13, and 14, end of this chapter). The gentleman wrote that he had accidently dumped a full pot of boiling water on his right foot. He immediately saw an emergency room physician, who said the burn was third-degree. The doctor removed dead tissue from Howard's foot, applied a prescription burn cream, and bandaged the foot. The patient was given instructions to repeat the cream and rebandage at home, and this he did. Four days after the incident and despite following the physicians instructions precisely , the burn victim's foot was so horribly swollen and painful that he went to a second doctor who basically repeated the instructions of the first doctor. Mr. Howard was now running a high fever in addition to being in agony from the burn.

At this point, the victim's sister suggested that he try an Aloe vera "jelly" product which she had used for burns. It took several days to procure the product by mail, during which time the swelling, pain, and fever increased. According to Mr. Howard, "I received this (the Aloe) at 4:00 PM Sept., 4, 1986. I cleaned the burn, applied (brand name of Aloe product deleted) at 6 PM. At 9:00 PM the swelling had disappeared and the temperature had subsided." Howard continued to use the Aloe product on his foot, which quickly and steadily improved, and says that the burn has completely healed but that the foot and bones remained tender for a while. Needless to say, Mr. Howard is now a firm believer in Aloe vera because he has seen with his own eyes what it can do.

Since he is not a sophisticated "scientist," he is perfectly willing to believe what he has seen with his own eyes and does not believe that what Aloe did for his burn is some sort of incredible coincidence. In other words, Mr. Howard didn't know (like so many physicians know because it is what they have been taught) that Aloe vera is "useless" for healing burns. He used Aloe for his burn after orthodox medicine had given him absolutely no relief. Since it worked very quickly and gave him demonstrable relief, he has no need to deny that it works. Or perhaps the reason Mr. Howard is happy to admit that Aloe worked is that he has no peer pressure or medical association to put pressure on him to deny what he has seen and experienced. All Mr. Howard had was a very badly burned foot for which he wanted help.

Many love their animals almost as deeply as they love their other family members. I met one such person, B.J. Butler, in 1985. After talking to her briefly, I could see she had a deep interest in Aloe vera and how it might be used to treat horses and others animals. Over the next few months, we had several long and detailed conversations about how to use Aloe vera.

A few mouths later, B.J. showed me some amazing pictures of the six-month old filly she had treated for an extremely serious hoof wound with concentrated Aloe vera "jelly." These pictures (See photos, Figures 15, 16, 17, and 18 end of this chapter) clearly demonstrate how quickly Aloe vera heals even serious injuries and that the healing time required is directly related to concentration of Aloe used and to the age and general health of the individual.

As the pictures clearly show, the animal in question accidentally cut off (apparently on a piece of sheetmetal), a large section of her left hind hoof and a large portion of the soft hoof bed. The wound wasn't discovered for approximately twenty-four hours, by which time it was covered with mud. B.J. thoroughly cleaned the wound with ordinary soap and water, packed it with "jelly," and then wrapped it to prevent the wound from getting dirty again. This procedure was repeated every other day although the wound was not washed. After the first application of Aloe, the filly was walking around in an apparently normal fashion and was not in pain. After thirty-two days, the fleshy wound was completely healed, the hair completely grown back, and the hoof was obviously regenerating. B.J continued treating the foot with "jelly" and within 72 days of the initial wound, the hoof itself was completely healed with no scarring and no limp. As of this writing, the horse is completely normal, running around and doing horse-things and is happy as "a clam." B.J. is definitely a believer in Aloe, and, of course, the horse didn't "know any better" and so got well in short order.

The speed at which Aloe vera will heal is, as we have said, directly related to the age and/or general health of the individual. This fact is illustrated by the experience of a then 70 year old friend named "Grandma" Ruby Leath. Mrs. Leath is a busy woman who runs a landmark museum-restaurant, known as the Old Plantation, in Medicine Park, Oklahoma. One day in 1985, Ruby was preparing to greet a large party of visitors to her business when she tripped on the front porch and fell against a large piece of driftwood which punctured her left leg. (See photos, Figures 19, 20, 21, and 22, end of this chapter) When Mrs. Leath finally was able to get to a doctor (some five hours after the injury), it took thirty stitches to close the wound. The doctor instructed Mrs. Leath to stay off her feet (which proves he didn't know her very well.) Within a few days, Mrs. Leath had pulled the stitches out and again saw the doctor who advised that a skin graft would be necessary. At this point, Mrs. Leath refused the skin graft and decided to treat the wound with Aloe vera. Quite frankly, this author must make it plain that the above chain of events was very unfortunate. As we have stated repeatedly, proper medical attention is imperative for the person who had suffered an injury. Mrs. Leath agrees that she should have followed the doctor's instructions which would have prevented reinjury to her leg. Open wounds which require stitches should always be seen and treated by a licensed physician.

Mrs. Leath has stated that she preferred using Aloe vera to undergoing a skin graft, an understandable preference. Unfortunately, Mrs. Leath used Aloe "jelly" on the wound in a rather irregular manner due to her extremely busy schedule. Furthermore, she suffers from varicose veins and poor circulation, which compounded her difficulties. Nevertheless, within one week, Mrs. Leath's leg began to heal noticeably, and she was encouraged to continue using the Aloe "jelly." After approximately one month of using "jelly," Mrs. Leath switched to a concentrated Aloe ointment. Her leg healed steadily over the next four months and today is entirely healed, although a slight scar remains. According to Mrs. Leath, this is "just another battle scar" which concerns her not at all.

I have also seen Aloe heal in a very dramatic manner. Probably the most spectacular example I have personally seen concerns a well- respected local businessman of my acquaintance, Lyle Ball. (See photos, Figures 23, 24, 25, 26, and 27, end of this chapter). In February, 1988, Lyle underwent a radical treatment for skin cancers which covered almost all of both his arms beginning from above his elbows and including the backs of both hands. The procedure was performed over a period of two to three weeks and involved chemically burning off the cancers (which were almost a solid mass.) Needless to say, Lyle was in extreme pain after the treatment. His physician gave him pain-killers and topical ointment, but Lyle said that the pain-killers did very little good. Lyle's wife knew something about Aloe vera and what it would do and suggested that Aloe might help with the pain and also help heal the chemical burns.

About 48 hours after undergoing the last treatment, Lyle began using a combination of the concentrated Aloe ointment and concentrated Aloe spray. He says he used both products "as needed" using pain as the criteria. According to Lyle, the extreme pain he felt was relieved almost immediately after he used the ointment and spray for the first time, and after one week the pain was eliminated.

As shown by the pictures, the burns on Mr. Ball's arms healed almost completely in <u>eleven </u>days! (Feb. 18 to Feb. 29, 1988.) As of this writing the skin on both Lyle's arms and hands is healthy and normal with little scar tissue.

The last story I will relate concerns a thirty-three year old man named Bill Butterworth, III, from whom I recently received an interesting letter. In February, 1987, a varicose vein ruptured in Bill's calf. (See photos, Figures 28, 29, 30, and 31, end of this chapter). The leg became "sore, hardened, and inflamed. Mr. Butterworth (for whatever reason) simply ignored the problem for three or four months. Only when the site of the vein "developed a small hole and began seeping blood" did Bill begin treating the wound with Hydrogen peroxide and Neosporin salve. Several more months went by in which "the sore kept getting bigger and so did the opening to the surface. It developed into an open crater-like wound because the skin around it was dying." It was also infected.

At this point, Bill saw a doctor who gave him an antibiotic ointment which temporarily stopped the wound from growing but did absolutely nothing to heal it. Several more months passed, and Butterworth saw another doctor who gave him the . same advice , and several more months passed.

Bill's wife now intervened and made him an appointment with a doctor of Internal Medicine. Tests were run, and the doctor recommended "wet to dry" dressings of saline solution. A surgeon was also called who likewise ran tests and said the veins in Bill's leg were "shot." The third doctor gave Butterworth more "wet to dry" dressing, special stockings, antibiotic pills, and told him to stay entirely off his feet. Need we say that this also went on for several months, with little improvement. Finally, Butterworth was given two alternatives by the surgeon: either go to the hospital for months of treatment, or go to the hospital for surgery to cut out the wound.

After receiving this bit of news, Mr. Butterworth took it upon himself to ask the doctor what he thought of using Aloe vera on the wound. According to Bill, the doctor said he thought Aloe products were "fine but was <u>not at liberty to tell me to use them or prescribe them. He (the doctor) said that is was "certainly worth a try and if it healed my wound, he</u>

wanted to know where to get it."

Butterworth immediately began to use two Aloe products on his leg--a spray and an ointment. According to his letter, Bill used the products for "less than four months and it (the wound) is almost healed." According to Bill, the physician was "very "impressed" by what the Aloe was able to do. He even asked for the address and phone number of the company which made the Aloe products!

There are a number of interesting elements to Bill Butterworth's experience. The most obvious point is that Aloe helped him after fourteen fruitless months of medical treatment. But what does it say about the state of American medicine when a licensed physician who thinks Aloe (as an alternative to treatment that is not working) is "fine" yet still is not "at liberty" to mention, much less prescribe, it for his patients? And remember the alternative for Bill Butterworth months in the hospital or surgery! Is it not truly a strange state of affairs, when the patient has to search around for a possible treatment because the doctor is not "at liberty" to recommend something which he thinks might work? The obvious question is. "What if, Bill Butterworth had never heard of Aloe vera?"

In the past, the sort of anecdotal evidence presented above has been subject to serious misuse. First, unscrupulous promoters of so-called Aloe vera (which often turns out to be either water or highly diluted Aloe) use such stories to promote their skimpy Aloe products. Their object is to make a fast buck by capitalizing on Aloe's name. Second, the medical and scientific community (with some exceptions) attack such evidence as untrustworthy because it lacks "control" apparatus to, supposedly, insure objectivity. Obviously, controlled studies are a valuable scientific tool, and this writer sincerely wishes that some brave physician would repeat several of the burn experiments which used Aloe as a healing agent (recounted elsewhere in this book) and insist that the results be made widely available both to his fellow doctors and to the general public. The doctor who undertakes such a study must, of course, be certain that he experiments with Aloe vera which contains sap.

As of this writing, there is at least one study being readied for publication which purports to show that Aloe sap heals burns. Needless to say, this writer is eagerly awaiting publication of the study. Yet, one wonders if, as in the past, this study will not simply be ignored by the powers-that-be, many of whom have completely closed their minds on the subject of Aloe vera.

The photos below show the use of Aloe vera after oral surgery. Dr. Bill Wolfe, D.D.S. states, "After removing the teeth and preforming an alveloplasty, I poured the gel inside the upper and lower dentures. The next day when the patient returned for routine adjustment, I discovered that there weren't any adjustments to be made! There had not been the swelling that usually occurs after such a procedure either. Now, I was excited!"

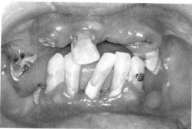

Fig. 1. "Immediate Denture-Previous to Surgery"

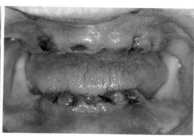

Fig. 2. "Immediately Post-Op"

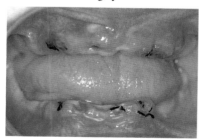

Fig. 3. "Twenty-Four Hours Post-Op

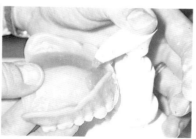

Fig. 4. " The Entire Inner Surface of the Denture is Covered with the Aloe Gel"

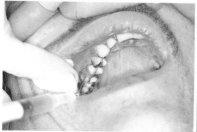

Fig. 5. "Aloe Irrigation post Periodontal Surgery"

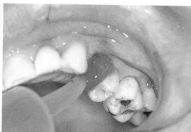

Fig. 6. "Aloe Flushing of a Fresh Extraction Site"

The case of Alfed Thompson:

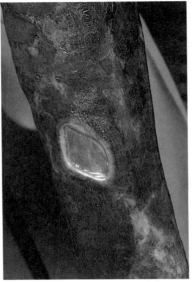

Fig.7. "Ulcer after one week."

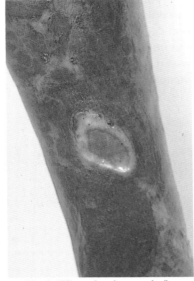

Fig. 8. "Ulcer after three weeks."

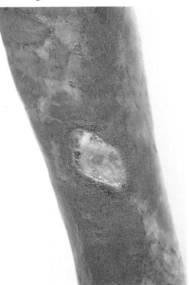

Fig. 9. "Ulcer after six weeks."

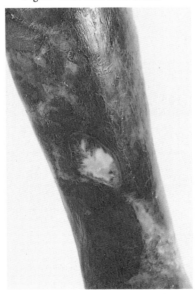

Fig. 10. "Ulcer after nine weeks".

The case of Johnny Howard:

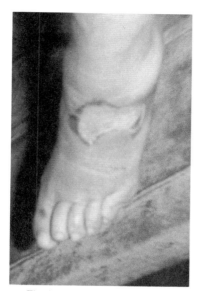

Fig. 11. "Burn prior to treatment."

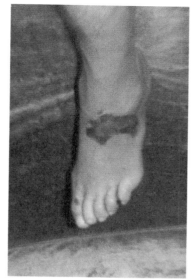

Fig. 12. " Burn after three days.."

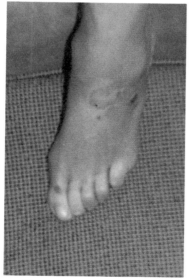

Fig. 13. "Burn after eight days."

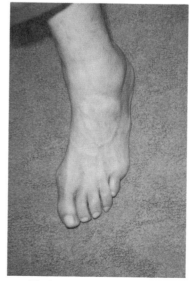

Fig. 14. "Burn after sixty days."

The injured hoof of a horse belonging to B.J. Butler:

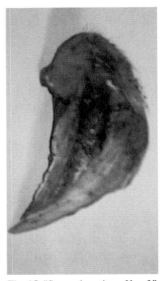

Fig. 15. "Severed portion of hoof."

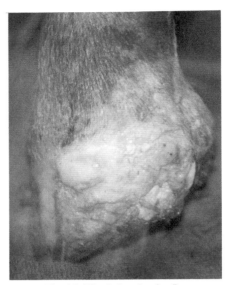

Fig. 16. "Hoof after cleaning."

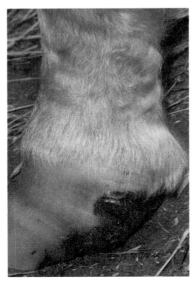

Fig. 17. "Hoof after 32 days."

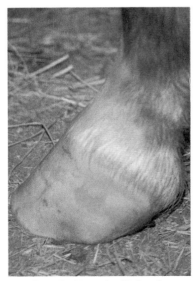

Fig. 18. "Hoof after 72 days."

The case of Ruby Leath:

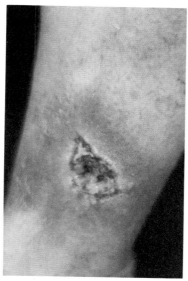

Fig. 19. "Injury prior to treatment."

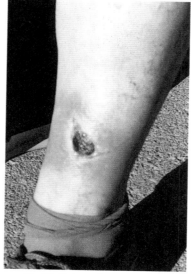

Fig. 20. "Injury after one week."

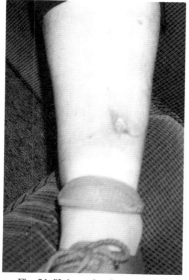

Fig. 21. "Injury after four months."

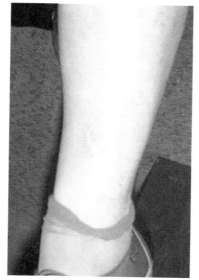

Fig. 22. "Injury after six months."

The case of Lyle Ball:

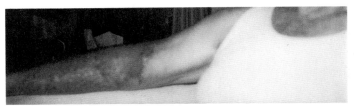

Fig. 23. "Chemical burn to right arm prior to treatment."

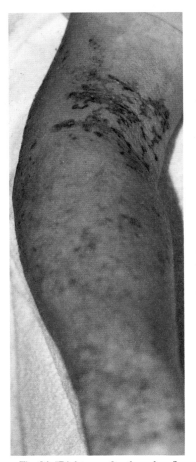

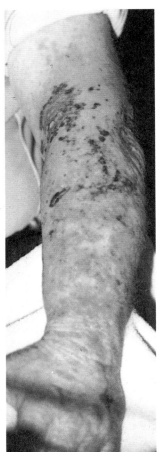

Fig. 24. "Right arm after three days."   Fig. 25. "Left arm after three days."

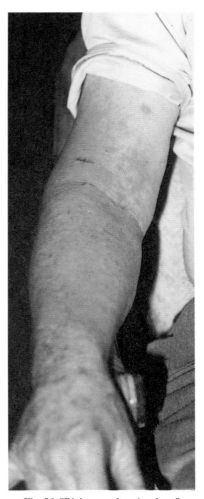

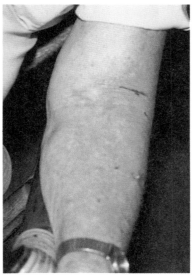

Fig. 26. "Right arm after nine days."

Fig. 27. "Left arm after nine days."

The case of Bill Butterworth, III:

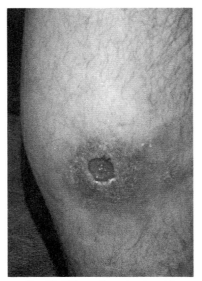

Fig. 28. "Ulcer prior to treatment."

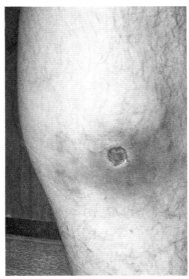

Fig. 29. "Ulcer after two weeks."

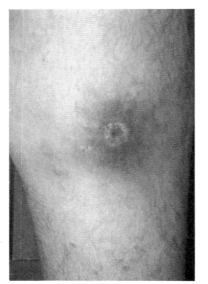

Fig. 30. "Ulcer after three months."

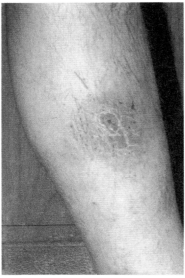

Fig. 31. "Ulcer after seven months."

CHAPTER FOURTEEN

ALOE VERA IN A NUT SHELL

The Plant

Genus: Aloe
Species: various
Family: Liliaceae (Lily)
Form: Succulent
Origin: Africa

Common Factors:

Numerous, fleshy green spear-shaped leaves with toothed edges growing in a rosette pattern from the upper portion of root or stem.

Single stem flower stalk, with two or more erect terminal spikes (candelabra shaped). Multiple stalks not unusual. Numerous tubular shaped flowers produced on top of terminal spikes.

Variations (natural):

Leaves of some varieties are a few inches in length, weighing a few ounces, while leaves of other varieties may exceed forty-eight inches, weighing several pounds. Leaf color, from light to dark green, with or without lighter spots.

Flower colors, yellow, red, and orange, (and possibly purple), and shades range from pastel to vibrant.

In tropical conditions mature plants of every variety bloom year round; in sub-tropic conditions, most mature plants bloom in the spring. House plants may never bloom.

Some species are stemless, with leaves growing at ground level, while others produce large stems (tree-like trunks).

Some species produce hard, thorn-like teeth, while others produce soft, pliable teeth. The spacing of teeth varies greatly.

Variations (environmental):

In tropical conditions the leaves of all species will reach maximum size of one to five pounds each, but in sub-tropic conditions leaf size is smaller in all varieties (from several ounces to three pounds.) Under poor growing conditions (lack of light, water, nutrients, and hard soil), all varieties are much smaller, and under long-term exposure to poor conditions, some varieties produce pencil-like leaves.

In tropical conditions stemless varieties grow to a height of four feet or more and stemmed varieties reach 30 feet or more; in sub-tropic conditions stemless varieties are smaller (one to three feet). Under poor conditions all varieties, stemmed or stemless, will be smaller.

NOTE: In our opinion the current confusion as to the number of species or varieties of Aloe vera is directly related to both natural and environmentally produced variations. These variations have led many to mis-identify the same species as being a new species, when in fact they are nothing more than the same plant which has adapted itself to its environment, like a chameleon changing colors to survive.

OTHER SCIENTIFIC NAMES:

Medical Aloes (plants that produce the sap) have been identified by various scientific names, both *official and **unofficial.

For example *Aloe vera Linne has been identified as Aloe perfolita var vera Linne, Aloe elongata Murry, Aloe vulgaris Lamarck, Aloe flava Pers., Aloe chinensis (Straud.), Aloe africana Miller, and others.

*Aloe perryi Baker has been identified as Aloe spicata Baker, Aloe africana Miller, Aloe perfoliata var vera Linne, Aloe soccotrina Lamarck, and others.

**Aloe ferox Miller has been identified as Aloe perfoliata ferox Ait., Aloe muricata Haw, Aloe horrida Haw, Aloe pseudoferox Salm-Dyck, Aloe subferox Spreng, Aloe africana Miller, Aloe ferou (Linn.), A. spicata (Thumb.), A. Africana, A. platylepia, and others.

NOTE: We do not know whether these names are accurately or inaccurately used, but in our opinion, they have done little to clarify the differences between sap producing Aloes and the hundreds of other species or varieties which have no recognized medical value. In fact, we believe they have only confused the public.

COMMON NAMES:

Aloe (the sap), when boiled down (to a black, dark brown, yellowish- brown, or reddish-brown mass, thick paste or liquid) has been identified by the commercial trade through the use of various common names.

For example, Aloe has been identified as Mocha Aloes or Jafferabad Aloes or Musambra Aloes *(India, mainly Bombay or Arabia), Uganda Aloes *(South Africa), Capey Barbados Aloes *(Caribbean), Zanzibar Aloes *(South Africa), Cabaline Aloes or Horse Aloes *(unknown), Natal Aloes *(South Africa), Lu Hui and Hsiang-tan, imported into China or Tibet *(unknown), and others. *(point of origin)

NOTE: As used here, the "s" on the word Aloes may be responsible for the belief that Aloe vera is referred to in the Bible (especially in the United States).

SCIENTIFIC NAME (Place of Origin)	ALSO KNOWN AS	NAMED BY (Flower Color)
*Aloe Vera Linne (North Africa, islands of Indian Ocean, Middle East)	*Aloe Barbadensis Miller (Commonly, Barbados Aloe, Islands of Barbados or Curacao Aloe, Islands of the Caribbean, i.e. Barbados and Curacao)	Carl Von Linne (Yellow)
*Aloe perri Baker (East of Africa, Cape Verde)	Socotrine aloe (From the island of Socotria, in the gulf of Aden, 150 miles east of Somalia)	Wykeham Perry (Unknown)
**Aloe ferox Miller (South of Africa)	Cape Aloe (Mainly South Africa)	Uknown (Red/Orange)

*Official varieties recognized by United States Parmacopia (U.S.P.) or British Pharmacopia (B.P.) because these plants produce Aloe (sap). **Unofficial varieties (not recognized by U.S.P. or by B.P., even though this variety also produces the sap are recognized by various cultures world wide.

A to Z

Historically, we find that Aloe vera has been used to treat human and animal medical problems from A to Z, and many more uses for the leaf have been suggested in contemporary literature:

-A-
Allergies, Abscesses, Abrasions, Asthma, Acne, Acid Indigestion, Allergic reactions, Anemia, Arterial insufficiency, Arthritis, Athlete's Foot

-B-
Bad breath, Burns, Boils, Bursitis, Baldness, Blisters/Blistering, Bruises, Bronchitis, Bloody scours in calves

-C-
Corneal ulcers, Contusions, Canker sores (Aphtous Ulcers), Cuts (lacerations), Cataracts, Chapped/chafed skin & lips, Coughs, Colds, Colitis, Carbuncles, Colic, Cradle Cap, Cystitis

-D-
Dermatitis, Dandruff, Dry Skin, Denture (gum) sores, Diaper Rash, Dish-pan Hands, Dysentery, Diabetes, Depression

-E-F-

Edema, Erysipelas, Epidermitis, Exanthema, Enteritis in fowl, Favus, Fissured nipples, Fever Blisters

-G-

Genital Herpes, Gingivitis, Glaucoma, Gangrene

-H-

Heat rash/prickly heat, Headache of all kinds, Hemorrhoid

-I-

Impetigo, Inflamed Joints, Insomnia, Ingrown toenails, Infertility due to invulatory cycles

-J-

Jaundice

-K-

Keratosis follocularis

-L-

Laxation, Leprosy, Laryngitis, Lupus

-M-

Multiple Sclerosis, Mastitis in dairy cattle, Mouth irritation,

Muscle cramps/strains

-N-
Nausea of all kinds

-O-
Onycolysis, Odor control of chronic ulcers, Oral disorders

-P-
Pin worms, Peptic and Duodenal ulcers, Psoriasis, Prostatitis, Poison Ivy/Oak

-R-
Razor burns, Radiation burns, Radiation dermatitis

-S-
Stings, Styes, Sprains, Senile moles, Sores of all kind, Seborrhea, Stretch marks, Sore throat

-T-
Tonsillitis, Tendonitis, Trachoma, Tuberculosis

-U-
Ulcerations of all kinds, Urticaria

-V-

Vaginitis, Venereal sores, Venous stasis, Varicose Veins

-W-

Wind burns, Wheal, Wounds of all kinds

-X-Y-Z

X-ray burns, Yeast Infections Zoster (shingles).

CONCLUSION

In 1983, I began to investigate an interesting puzzle--why Aloe vera works! Today, if a friend, neighbor, or even a physician asks me why it works, I tell them it works because the Aloe vera plant produces at least 6 antiseptic agents: Lupeol, salicylic acid, urea nitrogen, cinnamonic acid, phenol, and sulfur. All of these substances are recognized as antiseptics because together they exhibit antimicrobiological activity. This explains why Aloe has the ability to eliminate many internal and external infections. Lupeol, salicylic acid and magnesium are also highly effective analgesics, and this explains why Aloe is an effective pain-killer.

Next, I say that Aloe vera contains at least three anti-inflammatory fatty acids (cholesterol, campesterol and B-sitosterol, all of which are plant sterols), and this explains why Aloe is such an effective treatment for burns, cuts, scrapes, and abrasions, as well as a treatment for rheumatoid arthritis, rheumatic fever, and ulcers of all kinds, both internal and external. The presence of fatty acids may explain why some have stated that Aloe is highly effective for many inflammatory conditions of the digestive system and many other internal organs, including the stomach, small intestine, colon, liver, kidney, pancreas. The presence of any one of of these fatty acids, especially B-sitosterol, explains why it is often reported that Aloe juice is an effective treatment of allergic reactions and acid indigestion, and why it helps, in association with a low fat diet, to lower harmful cholesterol levels.

If the SYNERGISTIC RELATIONSHIP between the elements found in the plant's sap, its gel and throughout the entire plant does not explain why Aloe works, then NOTHING DOES! All of which explains why "Across Time" lay persons and physicians alike, have proclaimed that Aloe vera has the ability to heal, alleviate, eliminate, or even cure a monumental list of human diseases and disorders and therefore truly deserves the name "Medicine Plant".

Odus M. Hennessee

ADDENDUM

Since 1972, I, like millions around the world, have experienced the many benefits that can be derived from the use of Aloe vera on a daily or regular basis. In 1983, after almost ten years of using Aloe vera, I was extremely disappointed when a close friend informed me that Aloe vera was not used on the body of Christ, as I had long believed.

Like many of you, I had been misinformed and had gone about the business of sharing my experience, promoting Aloe vera by saying, "If it's good enough for Jesus, it's good enough for me."

The shock of discovering the truth led to the research which is presented here. There were other surprises to come. For instance, when this investigation began, it was intended to prove that the clear inner part of the leaf, Aloe vera gel, was responsible for the many benefits of the plant.

However, after less than two months of using the gel, I began to understand that the gel alone did not possess the ability to heal. What started out to be a short-term project has turned into almost six years of intensive investigation, research, work, and searching for the truth.

While plowing through a mountain of medical papers and other documents, most of which are original sources, numbering into the thousands, I began to understand that the problem with Aloe vera was that the information that was available had been divided out to the public in small pieces by those who appear to be more interested in selling an image than in investigating and presenting the facts; and that no one had ever challenged the confusion thus created. I discovered that much of what had been published by the Aloe industry was nothing more than what we in the United States would like Aloe vera to be, and not what it truly is.

Even though I started out to prove that Aloe vera that looked good, smelled good, and even tasted good would, in fact, heal, I finally came to the conclusion that if the truth were to be told, it must include the good, the bad and the ugly.

It is my hope that this book will inform, enlighten, and even entertain the medical professional and the lay person alike. But, more importantly, it is my intention that this work will shed the light of understanding on one of God's creations. It is my dream that this book will help all to understand that Aloe vera is a little myth and even some magic to those who believe; however in the final analysis, it is medicine to those who understand the plant, its properties, and why and how it works.

Odus M. Hennessee

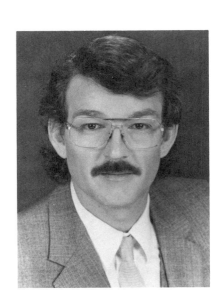

BIOGRAPHY

ODUS M. HENNESSEE

Odus M. Hennessee, a 40-year-old Oklahoma native and a 1972 graduate of Oklahoma State University School of Technical Training, is President of Cosmetic Specialty Labs, Inc., and Dream Valley Farm, both headquartered in Lawton, Oklahoma. Hennessee is also an inventor, and in association with two of his colleagues, introduced the Thermassage, a personal dry sauna thermal massage concept in 1988; he presently serves on the board of directors of Thermassage, Inc. He has been a licensed instructor of Cosmetology in the state of Oklahoma, since 1970.

His experience and expertise in many fields have helped make Cosmetic Specialty Labs, Inc. the largest wholesale private label manufacturer in the United States of Aloe-based personal care products including skin care, hair care, body care, and health care items. In 1981 he was instrumental in establishing Dream Valley Farm, and today it is the only greenhouse grower of Aloe vera in North America.

Born November 3, 1948 in Lawton, Oklahoma, Hennessee first experienced the benefits of Aloe vera in 1973, and because that experience he has devoted most of his time since 1983 to his pursuit of the truth about the plant. His analytical quest has resulted in a treasury of information about this plant commonly used as a home remedy around the world.

In his search, Hennessee turned to history, science and medicine to establish the validity of his long-held theory that the plant's active medical agents are mainly confined in the sap, but its total therapeutic value can only be achieved by using all three parts of the plant..

Due to his work, today Hennessee is a recognized authority on the subject. As a graduate of Dale Carnegie Sales Course and as a Sales Talk Champion, he is commanding and eloquent speaker, conducting seminars throughout the world...seminars which have done much to help educate others everywhere, not only about the virtues of Aloe vera, but also the use of plants in general for their health-giving properties.

Today, that search has led Hennessee to the forefront of his field. Hennessee believes that Aloe vera in cosmetics provides much more than just a cover-up for skin problems; he believes that it truly provides benefits which make our skin healthier, not just more attractive. Through his experience, he knows that the proper use of natural ingredients like Aloe vera in personal care products can make them more valuable to good health and well being.

After almost 20 years of experience in the personal care industry, Hennessee realizes that we have only begun to tap the ultimate potential of what proper personal care can achieve. He has learned realistically that despite his work and that of thousands of others, the investigation of the vast ability of plants to help heal our ills has only begun. As he puts it, the work is not done; it has only begun.

BILL R. COOK

Bill R. Cook, recipient of nearly 100 top awards in writing and photography, is a 1955 graduate of the University of Oklahoma. Cook's accomplishments in many fields have been noted in Who's Who, Who's Who In The West, Who's Who Among American Artists and Writers, and other biographical works.

As a journalist, Bill has authored short stories, articles, and papers on a wide range of subjects, and his photographs have been hung by major art galleries throughout the United States and in the White House, and several have been exhibited by royalty in England, Europe, and Africa.

Posts held include Hollywood picture editor, executive editor of three large publishing houses, producer of a television series, movie director and producer, magazine and newspaper publisher, and owner of a photography studio in Hollywood. He has served as corporate consultant and communications officer for a number of major cosmetic houses, and in 1970 he launched his own fragrance, cosmetic, and nutritional supplements company. From 1975 to 1986, he served as president and chairman of the board of Cook Communications, a California based communications agency.

Bill holds a black belt in judo, is a sponsor of the Olympiad of the Arts, and has headed committees in organizations including Kiwanis, Optimist Club, Jaycees, Y.M.C.A., United Fund, Cancer Association, and Knife and Fork Club. He has also been a member of Sigma Delta Chi, Pe Et Society, Sigma Theta Epsilon, International Grapho-Analysis Society, National Press Association, Peace Officer's Association, National Association, Inter-Religious Council, University of Oklahoma Alumni Association, University of Oklahoma

Alumni Development Fund, and University of Oklahoma Century Club.

As an accredited therapist and metaphysician, Bill assisted in the founding of seminar schools and as a platform speaker has conducted seminars in the United States, Canada, Africa, South Africa, Mozambique, and Swaziland.

Cook's interest in herbs as alternative treatment for human diseases resulted in his return to Oklahoma. His search led to a meeting with Edna M. Hennessee and Odus M. Hennessee. Subsequently, Bill joined forces with Odus in the writing of a book more than six years--a true labor of love--Myth, Magic, Medicine, Aloe vera Across Time.

BIBLIOGRAPHY

Abraham, Z. and Prasad, P.N. (1979) Occurrence of triploidy in *Aloe vera* Tourn. ex Linn. *Current Science* 48, 1001-1002.

Aleshkina, J.A. and Rostotskii, B.K. (1957) An Aloe Emulsion - a new medicinal preparation. *Meditsinskaya Promyshlennost'*, USSR 11, 54-55.

Al-Kindi, (1966) *The Medical Formulary or Agrabadhin of Al-Kindi,* translated with a study of its Materia Medica by Martin Levey.

Anderson, B.C. (1983) *Aloe vera juice: A veterinary medicament?* The Compendium on Continuing Education for the Practising Veterinarian 5, S364-S368.

Anton, R. and Haag-Berrurier, M. (1980) Therapeutic use of natural anthraquinone for other than laxative action. *Pharmacology* 20 (suppl. 1)104-112.

Ashley, F.L., O'Loughlin, B.J., Peterson, R., Fernandez, L., Stein, H. and Schwartz, A.N. (1957) The use of Aloe vera in the treatment of thermal and irradiation burns in laboratory animals and humans. *Plastic and Reconstructive Surgery, 20,* 383-396.

Ashleye, A.D. (1983) Applying heat during processing the commercial Aloe vera gel. *Erde International 1,* 40-44.

Bader, S., Carinelli, L., Cozzi, R. and Cozzoli, O. (1981) Natural hydroxyanthracenic polyglycosides as sun screens. *Cosmetic and Toiletries 96,* 67-74.

Barnes, T.C. (1947) The healing action of extracts of Aloe vera leaf on abrasions of human skin. *American Journal of Botany, 34,* 597.

Baruzzi, M.C. and Rovesti, P. (1971) Ricerche sull'azione cutanea del succo di Aloe vera L. Rivista Italiana Essenze Profumi Piante Officinali Aromi Saponi Cosmetici Aerosol 52, 37-39.

Batchelder, H.T. (1964) *Aloe vera Herbarist 30*, 25-29.

Beaumont, J., Reynolds, T. and Vaughan, J.G. (1984) Homonataloin in Aloe species. *Planta Medica 50*, 505-508.

Beccari, E. (1941) The pharmacology of the anthraquinone drugs, studied on the intestine "in situ" IV. the intestional behavior and the action of Aloe, *Arch. farmacol sper. 71*, 89-103.

Bland, J. Ph.D., (1985) Linus Pauling Institute of Science & Medicine, Palo Alto, CA., *Prevention Magazine,* Effect of Orally Consumed Aloe Vera Juice on Gastrointestinal Function in Normal Humans.

Blitz, J.J., Smith, J.W. and Gerard, J.R. (1963) Aloe vera gel in peptic ulcer therapy: preliminary report. *Journal of the American Osteopathic Association 62*, 731-735.

Bouchey, G.D. and Gjerstad, G. (1969) Chemical studies of Aloe vera juice. *Quarterly Journal of Crude Drug Research 9*, 1445-1453.

Bouchey, G.D. and Gjerstad, G. (1969), *Quarterly Journal of Crude Drug Research, Vol. 964*, chemical studies of Aloe vera juice II, inorganic ingredients.

Bovik, E.G. (1966) Aloe vera. Panacea or old wives' tales? Texas Dental Journal 84, 13-16.

Brandham, P.E. (1985) Jodrell Laboratory, *Royal Botanic Gardens*, Kew, Surrey, U.K. Personal communication.

Brasher, W.J., Zimmermann, E.R. and Collings, C.K. (1969) The effects of prednisolone, indomethacin and Aloe vera gel on tissue culture cells. Oral Surgery, *Oral Medicine & Oral Pathology 27*, 122-128.

Bruce, W.G.G. (1967) Investigations of the antibacterial activity in the Aloe. *South African Medical Journal 41*, 984.

Bruce, W.G.G. (1975) Medicinal properties in the Aloe. *Excelsa 5*, 57-68.

Capasso, F., Mascolo, N., Autore, G. and Duraccio, M.R. (1983) Effect of indomethacin on aloin and 1,8 dioxianthraquinone-induced production of prostaglandins in rat isolated colon. *Prostaglandins 26*, 557-562.

Cera, L.M., Heggers, J.P., Robson, M.C. and Hagstrom, W.J. (1980) The therapeutic efficacy of Aloe vera cream in thermal injuries: two case reports. *Journal of the American Animal Hospital Association 16*, 768-772.

Cera, L.M. Heggers, J.P., Hagstrom, W.J. and Robson, M.C. (1982) Therapeutic protocol for thermally injured animals and its successful use in an extensively burned Rhesus monkey. *Journal of the American Animal Hospital Association 18*, 633-638.

Cheney, R.H. (1970) Aloe drug in human therapy. *Quarterly Journal of Crude Drug Research 10*, 1523-1530.

Chinese Materia Vegetable Kingdom, revised from Dr. Frederick Porter Smith's work by Rev. G.A. Stuart, M.D., (1928 and 1932).

Chopra, R.N. and Ghosh, N.N. (1938) Chemische Untersuchung der indischen Aloearten Aloe Vera, Aloe India, Boyle. *Archiv der Pharmazie 276*, 348-350.

Coats, B.C. (1979) The Silent Healer: a Modern Study of Aloe vera. Bill C. Coats, P.O. Box 402 66, Garland, Texas.

Cole, H.N. and Chen, K.K. (1943) Aloe vera in oriental dermatology. *Archives of Dermatology and Syphilology 47*, 250.

Collins, C.E. and Collins, C. (1935) Roentgen dermatitis treated with fresh whole leaf of Aloe vera. *American Journal of Roentgenology 33*, 396-397.

Collins, C.E. M.D., (1935) *Vol. 57 No. 6 June, The Radiological Review and Chicago Medical Recorder,* Alvagel As A Therapeutic Agent In The Treatment of Roentgen and Radium Burns.

Crewe, J.E. (1937) The external use of Aloes. *Minnesota Medicine 20,* 670-673.

Crewe, J.E. (1939) Aloes in the treatment of burns and scalds. *Minnesota Medicine 22,* 538-539.

Crosswhite, F.S. and Crosswhite, C.D. (1984) Aloe vera, plant symbolism and the threshing floor. *Desert Plants 6,* 43-50.

Cutak, L. (1937) Aloe vera as a remedy for burns. *Missouri Botanical Garden Bulletin 25,* 169-174.

D'Amico, M.L., investigation of the presence of substances having antibiotic action in the higher plants, (1950) Lab. Inverni e Della Beffa, Milan, Italy.

Dastur, J.F. (1962) Aloe barbadensis Mill. In: *Medicinal Plants of India and Pakistan.* D.B. Taraporevala Sons & Co. Private Ltd., Bombay, pp. 16-17.

Diez-Martinez, S.D. (1981) *La Zabila, Communicado No. 46* sobre recursos bioticos potenciales del pais. INIREB, Mexico.

Fairbairn, J.W. (1952) Recent advances in the knowledge of the drugs containing anthracene derivatives. *Pharmaceutisch Weekblad 87,* 679-683.

Fairbairn, J.W. and Simic, S., *the journal of pharmacy and pharmacology V. 15,* (1963) the quantitative conversion of barbaloin to aloe-emodin and its application to the evaluation of Aloes november 19, 1962 from the department of pharmacognosy school of pharmacy, university of london, brunswick Square, London, W.CA

Fairbairn, J.W. (1964) The anthracene derivatives of medicinal plants. *Lloydia 27,* 79-87.

Farkas, A. (1963) Topical medicament including polyuronide derived from Aloe. US Patent 3, 103, 466.

Chemical Abstracts 60, 378g-379a.

Feil, C. (1980) Aloe cosmetics. *Bestways (USA). August, 1980*, p. 108.

Filatov, V.P., *American Review of Soviet Medicine*, August (1945), tissue therapy in cutaneous leishmaniasis.

Fine, A.F. and Brown, S. (1938) Cultivation and clinical application of Aloe vera leaf. *Radiology 31*, 735-736.

Flagg, J. (1959) Aloe vera gel in dermatological preparations. *American Perfumer and Aromatics 74*, 27-28 61.

Fly. L.B. and Kiem, I. (1963) Tests of Aloe vera for antibiotic activity. *Economic Botany 17*, 46-49.

Foster, G.B. (1961) First aid plant. *The Herb Grower 14*, 16-23.

Foster, G.B. (1965) Aloe again. *Garden Journal,* New York Botanical Garden 15, 239-240.

Foster, G.B. (1973) *Herbs for Every Garden*, 2nd edn. E.P. Dutton & Co., N. York City, pp. 96-99.

Fujita, K., Teradaira, R. and Nagatsu, T. (1976) Bradykinase activity of aloe extract. *Biochemical Pharmacology 25*, 205.

Fujita, K., Suzuki, I., Ochiai, J., Shinpo, J., Inoue, S. and Saito, H. (1978) Specific reaction of aloe extract with serum proteins of various animals. *Experientia 34*, 523-524.

Fujita, K., Ito, S., Teradaira, R. and Beppu, H. (1979) Properties of a carboxypeptidase from aloe. *Biochemical Pharmacology 28*, 1261-1262.

Galban, E.S. (1952) Florida herbs and plants. *Herbarist 18*, 16-23.

Gates, G. (1975) Aloe vera - my favourite plant. American Horticulturalist 54, 37.

Gjerstad, G. (1969) An appraisal of the Aloe vera juice. *American Perfumer and Cosmetics 84*, 43-46.

Gjerstad, G. (1971) Chemical studies of Aloe vera juice - I:

Amino acid analysis, *Advancing Frontiers of Plant Sciences 28*, 311-315.

Gjerstad, G. and Riner, T.D. (1968) Current status of Aloe as a cure-all. *American Journal of Pharmacy 140,* 58-64.

Goff, S. and Levenstein, I. (1964) Measuring the effects of topical preparations upon the healing of skin wounds. *Journal of the Society of Cosmetic Chemists 15,* 509-518.

Goldberg, H.C. (1944) The Aloe vera plant. *Archives of Dermatology and Syphilology 49,* 46.

Gottshall, R.Y., Lucas, E.H., Lickfeldt, A. and Roberts, J.M. (1949) The occurrence of antibacterial substances active against Mycobacterium tuberculosis in seed plants. *Journal of Clinical Investigation 28,* 920-923.

Gowda, D.C., Neelisiddaiah, B. and Anjaneyalu, Y.V. (1979) Structural studies of polysaccharides from Aloe vera. *Carbohydrate Research 72,* 201-205.

Grieve, M., (1971) *A Modern Herbal Vol. 1.* Dover Books.

Grindlay, D. (1985a) Medical use of Aloe vera. *General Practitioner (London),* Friday June 14th.

Grindlay, D. (1985b) Aloe vera. The Garden, *Journal of the Royal Horticultural Society 110,* 534-535.

Gunther, R.T. (1934) *The Greek Herbal of Dioscorides.* Oxford University Press, Oxford.

Gupta, R.A., Singh, B.N. and Singh, R.N. (1981) Preliminary study on certain vedanasthapana (analgesic) drugs. *Journal of Scientific Research in Plants and Medicines 2,* 110-112.

Harding T.B.C. (1979) Aloes of the world: A checklist, index and code. *Excelsa 9,* 57-94.

Heggers, J.P. and Robson, M.C. (1983) Prostaglandins and thromboxanes. In: Ninnemann, J.L. (Ed.), *Traumatic Injury. Infection and Other Immunological Sequelae.* University Park Press, Baltimore pp. 79-102.

Heggers, J.P., Pineless, G.R. and Robson, M.C. (1979) Dermaide Aloe/Aloe vera gel: Comparison of the antimicrobial effects. *Journal of the American Medical Technologist 41*, 293-294.

Heinerman, J. (1982) Aloe vera, the divine healer, In: *Aloe vera, jojoba and yucca*. Keats Publishing Inc., New Canaan, Connecticut, pp. 1-11.

Henry, R. (1979) An updated review of aloe vera. *Cosmetics and Toiletries 94*, 42-50.

Hirata, T. and Suga, T. (1977) Biologically active constituents of leaves and roots of Aloe arborescens var. natalensis. *Zeitschrift fur Naturforschung 32*, 731-734.

Hodge, W.H. (1953) The drug Aloes of commerce, with special reference to the Cape species. *Economic Botany 7*, 99-129.

Hoffenberg, P. (1979) Aloe Vera. Eine alte Heilpflanze - neu fur die Kosmetik. *Seifen, Ole, Fette, Wachse 105*, 499-502.

Horn, C.L. (1941) Botanical science helps to develop a new relief for human suffering. *Journal of the New York Botanical Garden 42*, 88-92.

Hranisavljevic-Jakovljevic, M. and Miljkovic-Stojanovic, J. (1981) Structural study of an acidic polysaccharide isolated from Aloe arborescens Mill. I. Periodate oxidation and partial acid hydrolysis. Glasnik Hemiskog Drustva. *Beograd. 46*, 269-273.

Ikawa, M. and Nieman, C., (1951) *archieves of biochemistry, further observations on the behavior of carbohydrates in seventy-nine percent sulfuric acid.*

Iller, Pepper and Wolfe, Bill, DD.s. (N.D.) A moment in dental operatory history.

Imanishi, K., Ishiguro, T., Saito, H. and Suzuki, I. (1981) Pharmacological studies on a plant lectin Aloctin A. I.

Growth inhibition of mouse methylcholanthrene-induced fibrosarcoma (Meth A) in ascites form by Aloctin A. *Experientia 37*, 1186-1187.

Jenkins, G.L. Ph.D., and Waldron, C.H. B.Sc., (1933) in *American Professional Pharmacist. Vol. 367*, Medicinal Agents in the Treatment of Burns.

Kameyama, S. and Shinho, M. (1980) Wound healing compositions from Aloe arborescens extracts. Japanese patent 79,151,113. *Chemical Abstracts 93*, 10375y.

Kent, C.M., (1979) *Aloe Vera*, arlington, virginia, pg. 14.

Khan, R.H. (1983) Investigating the amino acid content of the exudate from the leaves of Aloe barbadensis (Aloe vera). *Erde International 1*, 19-25.

Koshioka, M., Koshioka, M., Takino, Y. and Suzuki, M. (1982) Studies on the evaluation of Aloe arborescens Mill. var. natalensis Berger and Aloe extract. *International Journal of Crude Drug Research 20*, 53-59.

Leung, A.Y. (1977) Aloe vera in cosmetics. *Drug & Cosmetic Industry 120*, 34-35/154-155.

Leung, A.Y. (1978) Aloe vera in cosmetics. *Excelsa 8*, 65-68.

Levene, T. (1983) "Medicine men hit town with cactus cure". *Sunday Times (London)* 24th July.

Lion Corp. (1981) Cosmetics for skin. Japanese patent 80,104,205. *Chemical Abstracts 94*, 20244b.

Lorenzetti, L.J., Salisbury, R., Beal, J.L. and Baldwin, J.N. (1964) Bacteriostatic property of Aloe vera, *Journal of Pharmaceutical Science 53*, 1287.

Loveman, A.B. (1937) Leaf of Aloe vera in treatment of Roentgen ray ulcers. *Archives of Dermatology and Syphilology 36*, 838-843.

Lowenthal, L.J.A. (1949) Species of Aloe (other than Aloe vera) in the treatment of Roentgen dermatitis. *The Journal* of *Investigative Dermatology 12,* 295-298.

Lushbaugh, C.C. and Hale, D.B. (1953) Experimental acute radiodermatitis following Beta radiation. V. Histopathological study of the mode of action of therapy with Aloe vera. *Cancer 6,* 690-698.

Lutomski, J. (1984) Aloe, Topfzierpflanze mit therapeutischer Wirkung. *Pharmazie in unserer Zeit, 13,* 172-176.

Mackee, G.M. (1938) *X-rays and Radium in the Treatment of Diseases of the Skin, 3rd edn.* Lea and Febiger, Philadelphia, pp. 319-320.

McCarthy, T.J. (1968) The metabolism of anthracene derivatives and organic acids in selected Aloe species. *Planta Medica 16,* 348-356.

McCarthy, T.J. (1971) Aloe research. *Aloe 9,* 20-23.

McCarthy, T.J. and van Rheede van Oudtshorn, M.C.B. (1966) The seasonal variation of aloin in leaf juice from *Aloe ferox* and *Aloe marlothii. Planta Medica 14,* 62-65.

Mandal, G. and Das, A. (1980a) Structure of the D-galactan isolated from Aloe barbadensis Miller. *Carbohydrate Research 86,* 247-257.

Mandal, G. and Das, A. (1980b) Structure of the glucomannan isolated from the leaves of Aloe barbadensis Miller. *Carbohydrate Research 87,* 249-256.

Mandal, G., Ghosh, R. and Das, A. (1983) Characterisation of polysaccharides of Aloe barbadensis Miller: Part III-Structure of acidic oligosaccharide. *Indian Journal of Chemistry 22B,* 890-893.

Mandeville, F.B. (1939) Aloe vera in the treatment of radiation ulcers of mucous membranes. *Radiology 32,* 598-599.

Mapp, R.K. and McCarthy, T.J. (1970) The assessment of purgative principles in Aloes. *Planta Medica 18,* 361-365.

Meadows, T.P. (1980) Aloe as a humectant in new skin preparations. *Cosmetics and Toiletries 95,* 51-56.

Morales, B.L. (N.D.) Aloe vera-the miracle plant. Reprint from "Lets Live" *Health in Mind and Body,* Los Angeles, California.

Moroni, P. (1982) Aloe in cosmetic formulations. *Cosmetic Technology September, 1982.* **Morrow, D.M., Rapaport, M.J. and Strick, R.A.** (1980) Hypersensitivity to Aloe. *Archives of Dermatology 116,* 1064-1065.

Morton, J.F. (1961) Folk uses and commercial exploitation of Aloe leaf pulp. *Economic Botany 15,* 311-319.

Morton, J.F. (1977) Aloe. In: *Major Medicinal Plants-Botany, Culture and Uses.* Charles C. Thomas, Springfield, Illinois, pp. 46-50.

Morton, J.F. (1981) *Atlas of Medicinal Plants of Middle America. Bahamas to Yucatan.* Charles C. Thomas, Springfield, Illinois, pp. 78-80.

Newton, L.E. (1979) In defence of the name Aloe vera. *The Cactus and Succulent Journal of Great Britain 41,* 29-30.

Nieberding, J.F. (1974) Ancients knew value of Aloe for bee stings. *American Bee Journal 114,* 15.

Nikolaeva, V.G. (1979) Plants used by people of the USSR for treatment of infected wounds. *Farmatsiya (Moscow) 28,* 46-49.

Norris, J., (1973) Aloe vera. The ancient wonder drug. *Garden Journal, New York Botanical Garden 23,* 172-173.

Northway, R.B. (1975) Experimental us of Aloe vera extract in clinical practice. *Veterinary Medicine/Small Animal Clinician 70,* 89.

Noskov, A.D. (1966) The treatment of periodontosis injections of aloe extract and their influence on the phosphorus-calcium metabolism. *Stomatologiya 45,* 13-15.

Nouri, Y. Mary, Christensen, Bernard, and Beals, Jack I., (1956), the effect of some selected surface- active agents on the extraction of Cape Aloe, *Journal of the American*

Pharmaceutical Association Vol 45 (6).

Ovanoviski, H. (1983) Aloin. *Erde International 1*, 34-36.

Ovodova, R.G., Lapchik, V.F. and Ovodov, Y.S.(1975) Polysaccharides in Aloe arborescens. *Khimija Prirodnykh Soedineii 11*, 3-5.

Panos, M.B. and Heimlich, J. (1980) *Homeopathic Medicine at Home*. J.P. Tarcher, Los Angeles.

Papyrus Ebers (1553-1550 B.C.)

Paulsen, B.S., Fagerheim, E. and Overbye, E. (1978)Structural studies of the polysaccharide from Aloe plicatilis Miller. *Carbohydrate Research 60*, 345-351.

Payne, J.M. (1970) *Tissue Response to Aloe vera Gel Following Periodontal Surgery*. Thesis submitted to Faculty of Baylor University in partial fulfilment of the requirements for the Degree of Master of Science.

Pederson, M. (1987) *Nutritional Herbology*.

Pendergrass, E.P. (1959) Effective use of juice from the aloe vera leaf in the treatment of radiation reactions with excellent results.

Penneys, N.S. (1982) Inhibition of arachidonic acid oxidation in vitro by vehicle components. *Acta Dermatovener (Stockholm) 62*, 59-61.

Pierce, R.F. (1983) Comparison between the nutritional contents of the aloe gel from conventionally and hydroponically grown plants. *Erde International 1*, 37-38.

Pliny the Elder (78 AD) *A Natural History*.

Powers, M.B., D.V.M., M.S., (1969) Research Coordinator, Toxicology Division, Hazelton Laboratories, Inc., a subsidiary of TRW, Inc., Falls Church, VA *Paper examines acute oral toxicity of stabilized Aloe Vera gel*.

Proserpio, G. (1976) Natural sunscreens: vegetable derivatives as sun screens and tanning agents. *Cosmetics and Toiletries 91*, 34-46.

Radjabi, F., Amar, C. and Vilkas, E. (1983) Structural studies of the glucomannan from Aloe vahombe. *Carbohydrate Research 116*, 166-170.

Radjabi-Nassab, F., Ramiliarison, C., Monneret, C. and Vilkas, E. (1984) Further studies of the glucomannan from Aloe vahombe (Liliaceae). II. Partial hydrolyses and NMR carbon-13 studie.. *s Biochimie 66*, 563-567.

Raine, T.J., London, M.D., Goluch, K., Heggers, J.P. and Robson, M.C. (1980) Antiprostaglandins and antithromboxanes for treatment of frostbite. *American College of Surgeons Surgical Forum 31*, 557-559.

Reynolds, G.W. (1950) *The Aloes of South Africa*. The Trustees of the Aloes of South Africa Book Fund, Johannesburg, South Africa.

Reynolds, G.W. (1966) *The Aloes of Tropical Africa and Madagascar*. The Trustees, The Aloes Book Fund, P.O. Box 234, Mbabane, Swaziland.

Reynolds, T. (1985) The compounds in Aloe leaf exudates: a review. *Botanical Journal of the Linnean Society 90*, 157-177.

Roboz, E. and Haagen-Smit, A.J. (1948) A mucilage from Aloe vera. *Journal of the American Chemical Society 70*, 3248-3249.

Robson, M.C., Heggers, J.P. and Pineless, G.R. (1979) Myth, magic, witchcraft, or fact? Aloe vera revisited. *American Burn Association Abstracts 31*, 65-66.

Robson, M.C., Heggers, J.P. and Hagstrom, W. J. (1982) Myth, magic, witchcraft, or fact? Aloe vera revisited. *Journal of Burn Care and Rehabilitation 3*, 157-163.

Rostotski, B.K., and Aleshkina, Ya. A., (1958) Aloe emulsion (used for the prevention and treatment of skin diseases, such as radiation injuries, kraurosis, dermatitis, exzema, psorsisas, neurodermititis, herpes, etc.) (U.S.S.R.)

Radjabi, F., Amar, C. and Vilkas, E. (1983) Structural studies of the glucomannan from Aloe vahombe. *Carbohydrate Research 116*, 166-170.

Radjabi-Nassab, F., Ramiliarison, C., Monneret, C. and Vilkas, E. (1984) Further studies of the glucomannan from Aloe vahombe (Liliaceae). II. Partial hydrolyses and NMR carbon-13 studie.. *s Biochimie 66*, 563-567.

Raine, T.J., London, M.D., Goluch, K., Heggers, J.P. and Robson, M.C. (1980) Antiprostaglandins and antithromboxanes for treatment of frostbite. *American College of Surgeons Surgical Forum 31*, 557-559.

Reynolds, G.W. (1950) *The Aloes of South Africa*. The Trustees of the Aloes of South Africa Book Fund, Johannesburg, South Africa.

Reynolds, G.W. (1966) *The Aloes of Tropical Africa and Madagascar*. The Trustees, The Aloes Book Fund, P.O. Box 234, Mbabane, Swaziland.

Reynolds, T. (1985) The compounds in Aloe leaf exudates: a review. *Botanical Journal of the Linnean Society 90*, 157-177.

Roboz, E. and Haagen-Smit, A.J. (1948) A mucilage from Aloe vera. *Journal of the American Chemical Society 70*, 3248-3249.

Robson, M.C., Heggers, J.P. and Pineless, G.R. (1979) Myth, magic, witchcraft, or fact? Aloe vera revisited. *American Burn Association Abstracts 31*, 65-66.

Robson, M.C., Heggers, J.P. and Hagstrom, W. J. (1982) Myth, magic, witchcraft, or fact? Aloe vera revisited. *Journal of Burn Care and Rehabilitation 3*, 157-163.

Rostotski, B.K., and Aleshkina, Ya. A., (1958) Aloe emulsion (used for the prevention and treatment of skin diseases, such as radiation injuries, kraurosis, dermatitis, exzema, psorsisas, neurodermititis, herpes, etc.) (U.S.S.R.)

Rovatti, B. and Brennan, R.J. (1959) Experimental thermal burns. *Industrial Medicine and Surgery 28*, 364-368.

Rowe, T.D. (1940) Effect of fresh *Aloe vera* jell in the treatment of third-degree Roentgen reactions on white rats. *Journal of the American Pharmaceutical Association 29*, 348-350.

Rowe, T.D. and Parks, L.M. (1941) Phytochemical study of Aloe vera leaf. *Journal of the American Pharmaceutical Association 30*, 262-266. ʹ

Rowe, T.D., Lovell, B.K. and Parks, L.M. (1941) Further observations on the use of Aloe vera leaf in the treatment of third-degree X-ray reactions. *Journal of the American Pharmaceutical Association 30*, 266-269.

Rubel, B.L. (1983) Possible mechanisms of the healing actions of Aloe gel. *Cosmetics and Toiletries 98*, 109-114.

Saito, S., Ishiguro, T., Imanishi, K. and Suzuki, I. (1982) Pharmacological studies on a plant lectin Aloctin A. II. Inhibitory effect of Aloctin A on experimental models of inflammation in rats. *Japanese Journal of Pharmacology 32*, 139-142.

Schenkel, B. and Vorherr, H. (1974) Non- prescription drugs during pregnancy: potential teratogenic and toxic effects upon embryo and fetus. *Journal of Reproductive Medicine 12*, 27-45.

Segal, A., Taylor, J.A. and Eoff, J.C. (1968) A reinvestigation of the polysaccharide material from Aloe vera mucilage. *Lloydia 31*, 423.

Ship, A.G. (1977) Is topical Aloe Vera plant mucus helpful in burn treatment? *Journal of the American Medical Association 238*, 1770.

Sims, R.M. and Zimmermann, E.R. (1969) report on effect of Aloe vera on growth of certain microrganisms., baylor college of dentistry, *dallas microb assay services vol 1* pp

230-233.

Skovsen, M.B. (1977) *Quotations from Medical Journals on Aloe Research*. Aloe Vera Research Institute, Cypress, California.

Soeda, M. (1969) Studies on the anti-tumour activity of Cape Aloe. *Journal of the Medical Society of Toho University, Japan 16*, 365-369.

Soeda, M., Fujiwara, M. and Otomo, M. (1964) Studies on the effect of Cape Aloe for irradiation leucopenia. *Nippon Acta Radiologica 24*, 1109-1112.

Soeda, M., Otomo, M., Ome, M. and Kawashima, K. (1966) Studies on anti-bacterial and anti-fungal activity of Cape Aloe. *Nippon Saikingaku Zasshi 21*, 609-614.

Solar, S., Zeller, H., Rasolofonirina, N., Coulanges, P., Ralamboranto, A.A. ,Andriatsimahavandy, A.A., Rakotovao, L.H. and LeDeaut, J.Y. (1979) Mise en evidence et etude des proprietes immunostimulantes d'un extrait isole et partiellement purifie a partir d'Aloe vahombe *Archives de l'Institut Pasteur de Madagascar 47*, 9- 39.

Spoerke, D.G. and Ekins, B.R. (1980) Aloe vera - fact or quackery. *Veterinary and Human Toxicology 22*, 418-424.

Stepanova, O.S., Prudnik, N.Z., Solov'eva, V.P., Golovchenko, G.A. Svischuk, A.A., Grinberg, B.G. Dubkova, O.M. and Kozak, S.A. (1977) Chemical composition and biological activity of dry Aloe leaves. *Fiziologicheski Aktivnye Veshchestva 9*, 94- 97.

Suga, T. and Hirata, T. (1983) The efficacy of the Aloe plant chemical constituents and biological activities. *Cosmetics and Toiletries 98*, 105-108.

Suga, T., Hirata, T., Koyama, F. and Murakami, E. (1974) The biosynthesis of aloenin in Aloe arborescens Mill. var. natalensis Berger. *Chemistry Letters 8*, 873-876.

Suzuki, I., Saito, H., Inoue, S., Migita, S. and Takahashi,

T. (1979) Purification and characterization of two lectins from Aloe arborescens Mill. *Journal of Biochemistry 85, 163- 171.*

Taylor-Donald, L. (1980) Aloe Vera, "The Wand of Heaven". *Bestways (USA), August, 1980.*

Taylor-Donald, L. (1980) A Runner's Guide to Discovering the secrets of the Aloe Vera plant. *Runner's World (USA), December, 1981.*

Tchou, M.T. (1943) Aloe vera (jelly leeks). *Archives of Dermatology and Syphilology 47,* 249.

Trease, G.E. and Evans, W.C. (1978) *Pharmacognosy, 11th edn.* Balliere Tindall, London.

Waller, G.R., Mangiafico, S. and Ritchey, C.R. (1978) A chemical investigation of Aloe barbadensis Miller. *Proceedings of the Oklahoma Academy of Science 58,* 69-76.

Waller, T.A. (N.D.) Aloe vera. *A publication of Vera Products Inc.,* Taos, New Mexico.

Watt, J.M. and Breyer-Brandwijk, M.G. (1962) *The Medicinal and Poisonous Plants of Southern and Eastern Africa, 2nd edn.* E. & S. Livingstone Ltd. Edinburgh and London, pp. 680-687.

Wheelwright, E.G., (1974) *Medicinal Plants and Their History.* Dover Books.

Winters, W.D., Benavides, R. and Clouse, W.J. (1981) Effects of Aloe extracts on human normal and tumour cells in vitro. *Economic Botany 35,* 89-95.

Wolfe, Dr. B., and Iller, P. (1988) *aloe vera an ancient plant for modern dentistry,*

Wood, J.R.I. (1983) The Aloes of the Yemen Arab Republic. *Kew Bulletin 38,* 13-31.

Wright, C.S. (1936) Aloe vera in the treatment of Roentgen ulcers and telangiectasis. *Journal of the American Medical Association 106,* 1363-1364.

Yagi, A., Makino, K., Nishioka, I. and Kuchino, Y. (1977) Aloe mannan, polysaccharide, from Aloe arborescens var. natalensis. *Planta Medica 31*, 17-20.

Yagi, A., Harada, N., Yamada, H., Iwadare, S. and Nishioka, I. (1982b) Antibradykinin active material in Aloe saponaria. *Journal of Pharmaceutical Sciences 71*, 1172-1174.

Yagi, A., Shibata, S., Nishioka, I., Iwadare, S. and Ishida, Y. (1982a) Cardiac stimulant action of constituents of Aloe saponaria. *Journal of Pharmaceutical Sciences 71*, 739-741.

Yagi, A., Hamada, K., Mihashi, K., Harad, N. and Nishioka, I. (1984) Structure determination of polysaccharides in Aloe saponaria (Hill,) Haw. (Liliaceae). *Journal of Pharmaceutical Sciences 73*, 62-65.

El Zawahry, M., Hegazy, M.R. and Helal, M. (1973) Use of Aloe in treating leg ulcers and dermatoses. *International Journal of Dermatology 12*, 68-73.